T0380716

Divine Feminine Handbook

Volume III

Extreme Feminine Self-Care

MARILYN PABON

BALBOA.PRESS
A DIVISION OF HAY HOUSE

Copyright © 2021 Marilyn Pabon.

All rights reserved. No part of this book may be used or reproduced by any means, graphic, electronic, or mechanical, including photocopying, recording, taping or by any information storage retrieval system without the written permission of the author except in the case of brief quotations embodied in critical articles and reviews.

Balboa Press books may be ordered through booksellers or by contacting:

Balboa Press
A Division of Hay House
1663 Liberty Drive
Bloomington, IN 47403
www.balboapress.com
844-682-1282

Because of the dynamic nature of the Internet, any web addresses or links contained in this book may have changed since publication and may no longer be valid. The views expressed in this work are solely those of the author and do not necessarily reflect the views of the publisher, and the publisher hereby disclaims any responsibility for them.

The author of this book does not dispense medical advice or prescribe the use of any technique as a form of treatment for physical, emotional, or medical problems without the advice of a physician, either directly or indirectly. The intent of the author is only to offer information of a general nature to help you in your quest for emotional and spiritual well-being. In the event you use any of the information in this book for yourself, which is your constitutional right, the author and the publisher assume no responsibility for your actions.

Any people depicted in stock imagery provided by Getty Images are models, and such images are being used for illustrative purposes only. Certain stock imagery © Getty Images.

Print information available on the last page.

Scripture quotations marked KJV are from the Holy Bible, King James Version (Authorized Version). First published in 1611. Quoted from the KJV Classic Reference Bible, Copyright © 1983 by The Zondervan Corporation.

ISBN: 978-1-9822-7253-1 (sc)
ISBN: 978-1-9822-7254-8 (e)

Balboa Press rev. date: 08/31/2021

INTRODUCTION

What is Extreme Feminine Self-care?

First of all, self-care does not imply that you drop all of your responsibilities and focus on yourself exclusively. It doesn't mean that you have to practice an unusually high number of "self-focused" activities. It does not mean that you hang with your friends several times a week.

Self-care is not the same thing as getting your needs met. Extreme self-care is more commonly understood as knowing how to recognize and react healthfully to your own and other's emotions. It also involves mindfulness. It suggests getting the right amount of sleep, eating well, regular exercise, and benefitting from encouraging and supportive relationships.

Extreme self-care encompasses self-care and is also about how well we treat others, it includes preparation and reflection. It includes caring for those closest to us. When they are hurt, we will feel it too.

Your goal may be to feel happier, more confident, be healthier, reduce unwanted feelings of stress, anxiety, or depression. Concern yourself with your goals but have an "ideal vision" for your future. Aim to achieve what's important to you such as a peaceful existence, love, and harmony and not merely money or material wealth as a substitution.

Through extreme self-care, we come to know ourselves. We learn to realize the power we have to cultivate how we think, examine our beliefs, expectations, the actions we take, and our impact on others. Ultimately, we learn our health, what we think and how we feel is in our control.

Extreme feminine self-care is defined differently by each person, but here are some good places to start:

- **Food**: Everyone knows what foods make them feel great and what foods make them feel awful. Eat what makes you feel great and notice know how often you have to eat.
- **Sleep:** Only need four hours, six hours, or eight hours a night? Make sure you get the sleep that makes you feel your best.
- **Exercise:** Some folks won't do anything unless they can get their class or their run in. Just move as much as you can.
- **Prayer, reflection, meditation:** Take time to simply tune in, stop the noise, and unplug.
- **Rest and relaxation:** Do whatever makes you feel replenished.
- **Connection time:** Spend time with loved ones, family, and friends not out of obligation, just because you adore them.
- **Fun:** Anything you can do that raises your spirits and makes you smile is fun. Have some every day.

Leading a fully engaged life begins with focus on your divine life's worth:

- Relationships matter more than anything; The secret to leading a fulfilling life
- Health determines the quality of your life; Exercise / Nutrition / Rest

- Work gives voice to your giftedness/talents; Live in your strengths
- Hobbies engage your energy beyond work; Take time to enjoy things away from work
- Learning animates your imagination; Have a passion for personal development
- Faith gives your life purpose; Allow Spirit to guide your way

Each of these areas requires intentional focus to nurture at the highest level. This is easier said than done. You have a great deal on your plate between your personal, family, and work obligations, so finding time to properly care for these key areas of extreme self-care can be challenging.

We all have the exact same amount of time. You have 24 hours to use everyday. How you utilize that 24, is an indication of your priorities.

You must prioritize and carve out time for taking care of yourself:

- Build a plan to accomplish your extreme self-care initiatives
- Document your ideal Vision in each of these key areas of self-care
- Assess the gap between your Vision and your current reality in each area
- Set short term and long term goals to move you from your current reality to your Vision
- Celebrate your successes of progress on a consistent basis

You are an angel who has come to earth to take on human form to be here in the dimension of slowed down time and space, to live within your own creation, see the results of your thoughts, actions and consciousness, to expand your soul. You brought all the tools you need with you. You are so much more than you think you are and have more power than you can imagine.

This is a call to action for you to remember who you are, to love yourself and take care of yourself on this journey of your soul. Your soul is also called your spirit, your higher-self, your inner goddess, an angel in human form, your true essence.

Your awakening is a remembrance and a call to come back to your divine self. To live from your heart and trust in your "knowing" that was planted in your heart before you came to earth. That voice inside of you is your inspiration (in spirit), also called your intuition, your subconscious, your higher-self, etc.

Return to who you were before the world got a hold of you and told you lies, before you bought into the old stories, before you lost your self-confidence and self-love. Just look at a baby or small child and see the joy they have for life, their spark, their self- confidence and self-love, go back to that.

Put health and self-care at the heart of everything and you will enjoy reaping the endless benefits during this time you spend on Mother Earth. Healing the physical body is the beginning of getting to the root of healing the whole being. Learning the wisdom of self-care from our Divine Feminine ancient foremothers will put us back in touch with our inner knowing, our divinity and purpose.

Divine Feminine Handbook is a four-book series:
Volume I: Overcoming Self-Doubt
Volume II: Unleash Your Inner Goddess
Volume III: Extreme Feminine Self-Care
Volume IV: Self-Reliance in a Changing World

CONTENTS

CHAPTER 1

Your Goddess Body, Mind & Spirit

"Body confidence is when you honor your body for being the home to an incredible soul." - Jessica Ortner

Our spirits are full of intelligence, energy, love and magic. Our physical bodies which house our magnificent spirits can be restrictive and cumbersome and susceptible to illness. Taking care of our physical bodies is as important as our spiritual well-being. Our physical health affects our mental and spiritual health, which makes it a top priority. Healing the physical body is the beginning of getting to the root of healing the whole being.

In this modern fast paced world, we have to consciously take care of our bodies. In today's environment there is no margin for error or neglect. Our bodies are complex organic living organisms, yet simple to care for. We have to feed them organic living food and clean water, as nature intended and as our ancient ancestors did, simple, but not as easy as it used to be.

Have you noticed that modern convenience has abandoned traditional foods? Most of what is available to eat today, whether from the market or restaurant, is either highly processed or made with ingredients that are themselves highly processed. What do we lose when we stop eating traditional foods? Our health.

Processed food has additives, food colorings, preservatives, artificial flavoring, chemicals, processed sugar, flour, refined salt, genetically modified organisms, hormones and antibiotics. All of which cause disease, acidity, mucus, inflammation, constipation and dullness of the mind. Although sickness and disease are prevalent in our world, having a healthy life is not impossible. Consciously and carefully choosing the food you eat and don't eat is not an alternative lifestyle, it is the natural and original lifestyle we need to return to for vibrant health. This should be non-negotiable.

We live in a toxic food culture. Most of the food we eat today is not really food but it is all we have known since we were born. Real food comes from Mother Earth; plants, trees, bushes, roots, vines, herbs and animals. Real food is still recognizable the way it grows and is found in nature. If your food comes in a can or box or drive through window it is not real food that your body can recognize or use. You would be shocked if you knew how many people don't know where real food comes from or how it grows; On a tree? A bush? A vine? Underground? They've never seen it.

Our ancient ancestors had to work harder to collect their food but they did not have to question their food choices like we do. They didn't have to worry or know anything about reading labels, pollution, chemicals, hormones, GMO's, fake food, or being gluttons.

"Eat food, not too much, mostly plants" is sound advice. If you eat food directly from nature you don't have to worry about calories, trans fat, saturated fat or salt. When you focus on real food, nutrients tend to take care of themselves. If you eat more fiber, less sugar and flour and real food, as it grows in nature, you will give your body what it needs to balance itself and your weight will balance out as well. Healthy eating is a long term lifestyle goal, not a temporary fad diet.

We do not have to forage for our food every day but we do need to make a meal plan for the week, shop for ingredients and do some food prepping at least one day a week to have healthy food choices quickly and easily available for the rest of the week. It is inconvenient but necessary. Our ancestors are looking down on us shaking their heads in disbelief that we think this is too much work.

Your Inner Goddess would make her food choices wisely and to her best interest, love herself and take care of herself inside and out and be very particular where her food comes from and how it is prepared.

Healthy eating isn't restrictive, it's healing. Your divine health is something worth fighting for and tending to. I have worked with many wealthy clients who can buy anything but they can't buy their health back. Their money and luxurious lifestyles are nothing to them without their health. Regardless of your age or your previous eating habits, it's never too late to change your diet or improve the way you feel and think.

The Body Can Heal and Repair Itself

"Foolish the doctor who despises the knowledge acquired by the ancients." - Hippocrates

In the Eighteenth Century, magic and mystery were replaced by reason and logic. Their thinking was; if it cannot be seen or measured or proved, it does not exist. The divine disappeared.

The physical became the only focus in the Nineteenth Century, and the mind and spirit were of no significance. With the emergence of surgery and antiseptics nature's healing arts were pushed aside again.

Today when we get sick we go to the doctor who gives us a chemical medicine for the symptom we are complaining about. Western doctors do not believe food is medicine, they do not believe the body can heal and repair itself without their intervention. They do not believe nature has cures and they do not believe in spiritual healing or anything they cannot prove with science or learn in medical school.

If a doctor diagnoses you with a disease or condition and tells you it doesn't matter what you eat, it is a lie! Medicine is not health care. Food is health care. Mother Nature is smart, she put medicine inside the food.

- Eat fruits for electricity.
- Eat vegetables for grounding.
- Eat herbs for healing.
- Eat nuts for building.

You Continually Make A New Body

Every 28 days your skin replaces itself. Your taste buds, every 2 weeks. Your liver, every 5 months. Your bones, every 10 years. Your body makes these new cells from the food you eat. You can make new cells the same as themselves, better than themselves or worse than themselves, depending on your food choices and the environment inside your body. Food contains messages that communicate with every cell of the body.

The body can heal and repair itself if you give it what it needs and you take away what is harming it. God, Spirit, Creator, the Universe, Nature, whatever you believe it is, created our bodies to heal and repair themselves and live to be about 100+ years if we take proper care of them. Nature's way of death is that we peacefully pass away in our sleep, in our home, when we are old and worn out. Very few people die so peacefully any more. Most people die in pain and suffering from one disease or another, or several at one time.

The secret to a vibrant long life is to eat the way our ancestors did, the way nature intended us to nourish and heal our bodies. The key to this secret, is to love yourself enough to take responsibility, learn how to take proper care of yourself and then do it!

When thinking of food choices, I am reminded of the funny words in one of Jimmy Buffet's songs Fruitcakes "She treats her body like a Temple, I treat mine like a tent". He obviously was dealing with a Divine Feminine and didn't know it.

Your body is the temple for your soul, the one and only vehicle you get for your adventurous earthly journey. If you have a sick, sluggish, slow, aching body your journey won't be very long or adventurous.

Our Ancestor's Diets

Our ancient ancestors, by no choice of their own;

- Lived off of the land as Mother Nature provided
- Ate with the seasons
- Naturally detoxified each season as the food changed
- Intermittently fasted when food was scarce
- They ate organic food
- And drank clean water
- They ate mostly plant food
- And used plant medicine
- They ate when they were hungry, maybe they grazed or ate once or twice a day
- They ate animals when they could catch them, but it was hard work as they didn't have sophisticated hunting equipment, high powered rifles with telescopes and vehicles to haul them back to the tribe. The Paleo Diet theory has finally been debunked by science and anthropologists, the ancients did not eat a ton of meat.

- They eventually learned how to preserve food through fermentation and dehydration
- They gathered seeds and planted crops
- They cooked with fire and made soups and porridge and bread and on occasion ate a little meat

As a result, the ancients were healthy, fast and strong and their bodies self-repaired quickly when needed.

Modern Diets

"If someone wishes for good health, one must first ask oneself if he is ready to do away with the reasons for his illness. Only then is it possible to help him." - Hippocrates

In today's world, most busy working people are looking for cheap fast food. When you insist on natural, organic, clean, wild caught and grass fed you are considered eccentric. When in fact it was the original lifestyle for most of the history of the world.

I've been called weird, cuckoo, eccentric and a heretic, all by men, go figure.

Most people are not willing or unable to grow their own food or return to cooking and preparing their own meals from scratch. Their lack of understanding about what they are eating when they buy fast food, processed food and most restaurant food, will destroy their health causing unnecessary man-made illness and disease. If most of the foods you eat are processed and not alive, you will become chronically deficient in the nutrients your body needs to regenerate itself.

Living in our world of plenty, our diets are far from optimal. We rarely miss a meal, usually snack in between meals and have late night treats. Our meals are super-sized and most people overeat without realizing it. We never go hungry, there is food available to us 24/7. As a result, we have inflammation, pain, mental imparity, depression, fatigue, digestive problems, and many self-imposed diseases.

The idea of eating 3 square meals a day came from the English colonizers who viewed the native Indians as wild animals and believed their own tradition of eating 3 square meals a day is what set them apart from the "savages". How arrogant and foolish they were, but their traditions lived on to haunt us and have become a standard practice.

It is imperative that we change our western eating habits to clean eating and eating less. Your stomach is the size of your clenched fist and you should never eat more than what would fill up that space. Most peoples stomachs are stretched out from eating too much but they will shrink back to normal size as you begin to eat less at each meal and the bonus is your appetite will shrink as well.

We also need to detoxify the poisons we have allowed into our bodies for so many years. If we don't clean up our diets and detoxify the impurities stuck inside, we will follow in the footsteps of most modern westerners who fall prey to sickness and disease and live their last years in pain and suffering or an early death.

When we are sick and in pain we cannot think clearly and don't always make the best choices for ourselves. Once again giving away our power to someone else to "fix" us or "save" us from our poor choices.

"We are an overfed and undernourished nation digging an early grave with our teeth..."
Ezra Taft Benson, Government Official

Poor health keeps you in the very dense, low vibrating energy of fear, anxiety and depression.

A Goddesses Ideal Healthy Weight

Most women want to lose or gain weight because they don't like how they look. When they don't like how they look they usually develop a poor body image and lower self-esteem. This negative energy develops blocks to losing or gaining weight. So we first must address body image as it is a piece of the puzzle to obtaining your ideal healthy weight.

Body Image

To be truly happy and free you have to feel comfortable in your own skin. We are a fabulous spirit housed inside a human body of flesh and bone which morphs many times from infancy to old age. Our body is not a solid structure, it is a miraculous process which is ongoing. We are made up of more energy than anything else and energy can be manipulated. Your body has an amazing capacity to correct itself. To begin this process you have to feel comfortable in your body, trust it, love and appreciate it before you help it to change. You need a connection with your body that isn't blocked by shame, anger, or guilt.

What Is Your Comfort Level With Your Body? How Do You Feel When:

- You look in a full length mirror?
- Try on clothes in a store?
- Wear a revealing bathing suit?
- Have your picture taken?
- Being looked at in public?
- Being seen nude by your spouse or lover?
- Undressing at the gym?
- Attempting physical challenges?
- Playing team sports?

- Dancing?
- Being touched physically?

Becoming aware of your body image discomforts, weather physical or emotional, puts you back in touch with your body so you can begin a plan for overcoming them. Try the following exercise.

1. Make your personal list of body image discomforts.
2. Choose one image of discomfort:

    - Imagine yourself in this uncomfortable situation, feel it emotionally and physically.
    - Notice the negative energy associated with this mental image.
    - Tune in and be with the energy. Relax. Don't freeze up or get tense.
    - Now see if you can make the image in your mind change to the image you desire.

Some items of discomfort will take longer to change than others depending on how strongly it is imprinted in your brain. As you imagine how you want to look and feel about a particular item of discomfort, attach your emotions and intention to the image you desire, as this will amplify your success.

The more often you do this exercise the more successful you will be in overcoming your discomforts and learn to love your Divine Feminine body. Your body loves you and believes what your mind tells it.

3. Work on each of your body image discomforts, one at a time. With all lists I find it best to choose the easiest item to change first and work my way up to the most difficult. You will have greater success with this plan rather than

first tackling the hardest thing to change. You will quit the whole exercise before you make any progress.

Don't give up, you will prevail. Writing your experiences and feelings in your journal allows the emotions and negative thoughts to leave your body and land on the page, where it is captured, freeing you from carrying it inside you any longer. This step is important for your healing and closure.

You must learn to love your body and accept it in spite of its imperfections, some of which you may or may not be able to change.

Now we can move on with our discussion of your personal ideal healthy weight. You may want to loose weight to look better, feel better about yourself, improve your health or all of these reasons, but have not been completely successful because it so hard to do!

Why Is Change So Hard?

Most of us can change what, when, and how much we eat for a little while. But once our newfound "willpower" runs out, we fall right back into old habits. Every single time!

Why is breaking up with destructive eating behaviors so hard to do?

It's complicated and primal, and it has everything to do with your brain trying to help you survive. Yes, even if the eating changes that you're trying to make will make you healthier. Deep within our brain lies a basic quest for survival, located in the reptilian brain. Food is key to our survival and it represents safety. So if someone (even you) starts messing around with your food, all bets are off. That's because any threat to your safety, whether real or perceived, evokes fear.

You Are a Cave Woman

You have the same body the prehistoric cave-woman had, evolution has not changed that. Your body is designed to protect you from the dangers in the prehistoric world, which would be; starvation, freezing and being eaten. For thousands of years our ancestors had to worry about these three things, as a result our bodies are very good at protecting us from them. Today most of us don't have to worry about these things but our bodies don't know that. Our bodies still function with the same ancient genetic coding that has protected us from the beginning of time.

If you lived in the prehistoric world and food was scarce and unpredictable, your body would hold on to all of the calories you didn't use for energy by turning them into fat and save it to be used for energy at a later time. This is the body's way of keeping you alive. The more fat you had on you the longer you could survive a famine.

If you lived in a climate of cold weather your body would slow down your metabolism to use as little energy as possible, so it could make fat to insulate your vital organs and keep you from freezing. Being fat could keep you alive.

If you lived in a land of man eating predators where you were at risk of being eaten, fat would no longer be your friend. In these circumstances your body would want to be thin because being thin would be your best chance of being fast and therefore safe. In this case being thin could save your life.

Our bodies can quickly determine how much fat would be the ideal amount in any living condition, quickly adjusting this ideal weight as circumstances change.

The stresses in modern life are different than in ancient times but the chemicals that stress induces are the exact same ones our ancestors produced when they were cold or hungry or afraid and the body reacts in the same way to save you.

We have all heard that stress makes us fat, now you know

why. Our bodies make us fat because they love us and are trying to protect us and save us from the dangers in the world.

You can now understand why diets don't work. When you restrict your calories your body perceives it as scarcity or starving and makes more fat to save you. When you try to force your body to lose weight you are violating your body's natural laws of preservation. You may initially lose weight on your diet but as soon as you quit, your body will self correct itself and make fat to save you from the next famine.

If you are currently carrying extra weight then your body believes it is not safe to lose the weight. When your body believes it is safe to be thin it will force you to lose the extra weight. When you learn to work with the body's natural laws rather than fight against them, weight loss will become automatic and inevitable.

Mental and Emotional Stress

Your body treats mental and emotional stress the same as if it were a physical stress, you are sending a message to the body that says "I am not safe". Your body is made to protect you, the only kind of threat it understands is physical. To your body, threat means you are being attacked, freezing or starving.

If you have a fear of not having enough money, the only resource the body understands is food, and it will interpret your fear of lack of money as fear of lack of food and a famine is coming, so it will stock up as much fat as it possibly can.

If you are staving for attention or staving for love or intimacy, the only starving your body understands is physical starvation, and will once again stock up on fat to save you.

Food As Love

Food also has a strong emotional pull. Part of our habits with food have been built within the reward pathways of our brain. Not just the reward of pleasure, but those representing connection, bonding, and even love. Food is not just food, it can mean so much more.

This is one more reason why self-love and self-care is so important. We cannot always rely on outside sources to love and comfort us, and food doesn't have to be detrimental to us.

Don't Lose Hope

As humans, as well as the ancient brain, we have a higher-level brain with the ability to plan, reason, and see things through to the end. Change is hard, and requires accepting that we won't return to the old ways. We may need to accept that we can no longer eat like we did when we were younger or healthier, or that more movement will need to be built into our lives on a daily basis. Instead of resisting these changes, we can welcome them as part of our evolving reality.

Long-term changes in our nutrition and mindset require practice and forming new habits. Take the long view, making small, incremental changes that build over time. For example, start by making one meal a bit healthier and add one day of exercise per week.

Beliefs

You are a powerful soul. Your body is your tool, it's job is to protect you and keep you alive. Your body believes what you tell it, it is your willing servant. Your beliefs have great power over your body.

There have been terminally ill patients who believed they would be healed and then they were. There have been patients who were told they had a potentially fatal disease and they believed they were going to die and then they did.

In Australia there is an Aboriginal practice thousands of years old called "pointing the stick or pointing the bone". One of the duties of the Shaman or medicine man was to settle communal disputes. If it was determined that someone deserved severe punishment the medicine man would point the sharp bone at the offender and tell them they were going to die. They believed it so strongly that they actually got sick and couldn't eat or drink and they died. The guilty person would sometimes try to run away and hide but the Shaman would hunt them down to "point the bone" at them, and sure enough they would die. It was such a common practice and accepted belief that Australia had to pass a law and tell them they could no longer "point the bone".

The point being that our beliefs can control our entire reality, in our world and our body. Why let old dysfunctional beliefs get in your way of losing weight or maintaining your ideal weight? You can use the power of your Divine Feminine beliefs to your advantage.

Positivity

If you can get into the habit of automatically thinking positively you will be able to cut 90% of the stress signals which makes your body believe you are not safe and need fat to protect you. Thoughts are habits and the more we think a certain way we reinforce those thinking habits. When you are a habitually positive thinker the stresses in your life don't affect you as much and therefore you generate fewer mental starvation signals. You are less likely to be fearful, angry or give power to negative beliefs.

Breathing Exercise

Begin by slowing your breath, breath normal but slower. Breath in to a count of six, breath out to a count of six. After six inhales put your hand on your heart and say "I am safe" while you continue to breath slowly. For the next six inhales tell yourself "I am safe". You will become calm, relieve stress and your heart rate will slow down.

When you are calm and safe you naturally breath slowly.

When you are stressed, fearful or in danger you breath fast. By slowing your breath with your hand on your heart and telling your heart you are safe, your ancient brain will believe it and not have a need to store fat or make more fat to keep you "safe".

Repeat this slow breathing exercise several times a day.

Visualization

Just as you can use pictures to communicate with someone who doesn't speak your language you can use pictures to communicate with your brain.

Symbols and pictures are the universal language everyone understands. It's no different communicating with your own body. If you create a visual image of a leaner version of yourself, your brain will understand and work to make it happen. When you create a visual image of exactly how you want to look you are basically programming yourself to look that way.

Vision Boards have been popular for many years because they are effective.

- Cut out pictures of bodies you want yours to look like and glue them on your vision board. You can also use pictures of yourself at your ideal weight if you have them.
- Put the board somewhere you will see it everyday and it will send the message to your subconscious this is what it is suppose to look like.
- Imagine how you will feel, how it would change your life and what you would be doing if you were at your ideal weight and add those images to your board.
- Look at your vision board several times a day to keep your goal in the front of your mind, and you will begin to believe you are going to look the way you are visualizing your body to be.

Imagery Exercise

There are many emotional matters interwoven in the obesity problem. This problem is experienced as a muted unhappiness connected with beliefs about scarcity in your life. Survival is the "issue" here, your ancient brain believes that scarcity could lead to starvation and death. If you feel deprived of "nourishment" and don't make your needs known openly, you react by overeating.

The following imagery exercise may help you sort out the emotional connection with your weight.

- Imagine yourself in a mirror, seeing yourself thinner, healthier and happier in there and then seeing yourself enter the mirror and merging with the image.
- Notice the sensations you experience. Say to yourself "This is me!" or "I love my body!" or "I love being alive!" Whatever you are saying, really feel it to be true.
- Each time you are about to eat, see this image you are becoming and remember the sensations you felt in your thinner body.
- Seeing this image of the thinner you in the mirror for several minutes reinforces your intention.
- When you sit down to eat, tell yourself the content of your meal that you are about to eat. Then tell your body to take exactly what it needs and to reject what it doesn't need.
- Do this at every meal.

Cave Woman VS Modern Woman

It is actually a good thing we still have our cave woman bodies. Our world is ever changing and unpredictable as we now face climate change, pandemics, pollution and dying soil, our adaptable cave woman bodies are what we and our future generations may need to keep us alive.

Stress

We are bombarded with constant noise, light pollution and unprecedented stress. Most people spend 90% of their time in buildings breathing recycled air, under artificial light, surrounded by radiation from electromagnetic frequencies from computers, cell phones, wifi, tv's, home appliances, and smart home devices. Many people can even go years without their bare feet actually touching or connecting to the earth because they wear rubber shoes when they go outside.

- Some people are uncomfortable with silence. They can't turn off the chatter in their minds, they always have on the TV or music or just talk to avoid silence.
- Some people are afraid of the dark and never turn out the lights.
- Some people have problems focusing, concentrating and meditating.
- Some people are constantly uptight, their nerves are shot and they blow up over minor things.
- Some people worry so much they can't sleep properly at night.

De-Stress, Relax and Unwind

The ancient Divine Feminine did not worry about being politically correct. She did not hold in her feelings or thoughts if someone was inappropriate to her, cruel or unkind to others, she called them out and put them in their place. She didn't hold in stress and suffer to be "nice" to someone else who wasn't being nice.

She did not take on more than she could handle and multitask to the point of exhaustion. She made sure everyone helped and did their fair share to contribute to the well-being of the family and community. She was not a martyr who allowed others to sit back and reap the rewards of her hard work.

The Divine Feminine did not try to be everything to everyone, she was the Goddess who was revered, respected and loved, not one to be used or taken advantage of.

Relax, slow down and take it easy once in a while. Its ok to do nothing sometimes. Your body needs to rest but your mind needs to rest even more. Stress is not only uncomfortable it creates disease and fat. We need to quiet our minds and stop the negative self talk and sense of overwhelm that stresses us out.

Take a Break and Enjoy a Cup of Tea

Matcha Green Tea: Traditional Japanese and Zen tea ceremonies use matcha tea for ceremonies that are symbolic of peace, harmony, and happiness. Matcha is a high-grade green tea powder that can have up to 15 times more nutrients than loose leaf green tea. It does have some caffeine, so if you're caffeine sensitive, or wanting to enjoy a tea ceremony in the evening, I'm including below a number of herbal teas that are the perfect choice for a spiritual tea ceremony.

Ginger Tea: Ginger is warming, widens blood vessels for increased circulation, and supports the immune system. The spicy energy of ginger tea is beautifully aligned with the energies of love, money, success, and power.

Chamomile Tea: Most often used to promote good sleep, chamomile has several amino acids that have a relaxing effect on the body. Energetically chamomile is relaxing and purifying.

Holy Basil or Tulsi Tea: Holy Basil is a great supplement for overall health and wellness. It's an adaptogen, which means that it brings balance and calm. Tulsi tea is energetically nourishing, cleansing, and works to cut through stress and promote peace. Tulsi tea also balances your energy and purifies the mind, body, and spirit.

Mint Tea: Mint includes a broad category of herbs, all known for their uplifting effect. It's another anti-inflammatory and is often used for colds, headaches, and nausea. Mint is clarifying, and can help you cut through illusion and call positive energy into your life.

Rooibos Tea: Rooibos is a delicious red tea. Its high in Vitamin C and is said to help fight disease and signs of aging. It has no natural caffeine and yet is naturally energizing and rejuvenating.

Take Relaxing Baths

- Hot water baths are excellent to cleanse your body as the warmer temperatures tend to kill all the germs that you are exposed to throughout the day. It is also helpful in maintaining better personal hygiene.
- They are extremely beneficial to relieve cold and cough as the hot water and steam tends to clear your airways and help in decongesting your nose and throat.
- They are also known to beat insomnia and sleep disorders and are excellent to induce sleep.
- Hot water baths are also known to relieve stress and fatigue and also help relax sore muscles. It has also been shown to improve the flexibility of muscles giving you a supple body.
- Studies have also shown that hot water showers reduce sugar levels in the body making them ideal for diabetics. This study showed that sugar levels of diabetics who

immersed themselves in hot water tubs for 20 – 30 minutes for three weeks, had reduced by 13%.

- Ideally, soaps available in the market should be avoided and organic products must be used, as the skin absorbs all the chemicals when it is exposed to soaps and detergents. It is also recommended that a good lotion or oil massage, after bathing, has tremendous health benefits as it improves your skin textures and revitalizes your muscles and nervous system. Bathing for too long should be avoided.
- The element of water is feminine. Soaking in a hot bath connects you with the flow of feminine energy. It encourages you to rest. And just be.

Pick out at least one of the Divine Feminine essential oils below. Treat yourself! Then schedule at least one spa bath per week.

Jasmine: Nicknamed "Queen of the Night", a beautiful, seductive fragrance that helps balance feminine energy.

Ylang Ylang: Restores self-love & self-confidence. It also enhances sexual energy.

Patchouli: A calming, sedating & relaxing oil.

Rose: Rose is the oil of the heart chakra. It possesses the highest frequency of all essential oils.

Prioritize Sleep

Restful sleep is critical for the body to detoxify and heal. If you are not sleeping, you will not detoxify. This means not only the ability to fall asleep, but also to stay asleep and achieve a restful REM state.

Boost up your self-care. Get into bed early. Focus on the must-do items on your to-do list. Take extra time to journal or meditate or simply relax, and notice the effects on your energy when you take that extra special time to feel better. You deserve it! Your body needs adequate sleep to rest, heal and repair and even to loose extra weight.

Listen to Your Favorite Music

Music is in our blood, it is in our DNA. During excavation works, archaeologists often find some remains of musical instruments. Scientists suspect that between 60,000 BC and 30,000 BC, at the time when people began to create art (wall paintings, clay figurines), they also started to generate sounds consciously.

We can logically deduce that the beginning of music came from naturally occurring sounds and rhythms. Body slaps, clapping, foot stomping, and other functions could be used to create patterns and repetition. Using voices to imitate animals and the sounds of nature led to the eventual creation of musical instruments to better reproduce those sounds. Logs, shells, and rocks could be made into rudimentary percussion instruments, while bones and sticks could be fashioned into whistles or flutes. The instruments most frequently found by archaeologists include various types of flutes, whistles and pipes made of wood or animal bones.

Drums aren't found often since they were made of animal skins and wood which have deteriorated in the earth. But there are many paintings, carvings and status showing the use of drums. The shape of the drum was vital to the circumstance in daily life. Hourglass shaped drums were used for entertainment purposes, while kettle drums made of pots were used in celebrations. Drums could be tuned to vary their pitch in a variety of ways, including using water or heat to loosen or tighten the drum head, respectively. Many cultures used drums in their religious ceremonies to ward off evil spirits and to please guardian deities. Mostly drums were used to accompany singing and dancing, a vital part of prehistoric and early civilization.

Listening to music can be entertaining and some research suggests that it might even make you healthier. Music can be a source of pleasure and contentment, but there are many other psychological benefits as well.

Research proves that when you listen to music you like, your brain releases dopamine, a "feel-good" neurotransmitter which biologically causes you to feel emotions like happiness, excitement, and joy.

Listening to music you enjoy decreases levels of the stress hormone cortisol in your body, which counteracts the effects of chronic stress. This is an important finding since stress causes 60% of all our illnesses and disease.

Music can decrease pain in intensive care patients and geriatric care patients, but the selection needs to be either classical pieces, meditative music, or songs of the patient's choosing, usually being songs of their youth. Bob Marely was right about this one; *listen to music you love to take your pain away.*

Stroke patients who listened to music they chose themselves for two hours a day had significantly improved recovery of cognitive function compared to those who listened to audio books or were given no listening material. Most of the music contained lyrics, which suggests that it's the combination of music and voice that bolstered the patients' auditory and verbal memory. Stroke is the number 5 cause of death in the United States. If you know someone who has suffered a stroke, bring their favorite songs as soon as you can. Listening to them can significantly ramp up their recuperation.

Research shows that taking music lessons predicts higher academic performance and IQ in young children. In one study,

6-year-olds who took keyboard or singing lessons in small groups for 36 weeks had significantly larger increases in IQ and standardized educational test results than children who took either drama lessons or no lessons. The singing group did the best. To help your children achieve academic excellence, encourage them to sing or learn to play an instrument.

Once again our ancient ancestors knew what our modern science has to prove to us. Plato had it right when he said, "*Music and rhythm find their way into the secret places of the soul.*"

To stay calm and healthy during a stressful day, turn on the radio. Be sure to sing along and tap your feet to the beat to get the maximum healing benefit.

Watch a Movie

Hands down, entertainment is the principal reason for the entire world watching movies. Among the foremost benefits of watching movies, one has to be its role as a stress buster. You don't need a shrink to tell you to go watch your favorite movies or the latest releases. You know it as well as anybody else what a good movie outing with friends or just one in the comforts of your home can prove to be. Whatever the genre, as long as you enjoy it a movie elevates your senses and refreshes you for a fresh dose of reality.

Movies are entertainment which creates laughter and happiness. And there's no doubt that it has immense influence over both mental and physical health.

Through movies, you can find new perspectives that will help you reflect on and change your attitude. The different perspectives you see in movies can change your mental schemas and push you to be more creative, flexible, and innovative. The qualities of different characters can inspire you to improve your strengths.

Read a Book

The Advantages of Reading Books:

- Reading Books Is A Distraction
- Reading Can Reduce Stress
- Reading Books Can Be Your Best Teacher
- Reading Makes You Smarter
- Reading Books Makes You Better
- Reading Books Boosts Your Confidence Levels
- Reading Improves Memory

Spend Time in Nature

No matter how tired you are, spending some time in nature can help you to charge your inner battery and you can get relaxed and rejuvenated.

You don't have to go camping or to a state or national park to enjoy nature. It can be a wooded park or a community park, it does not matter as long as you can breathe the fresh air, feel the cold air rippling over your skin, hear the soft sound made by green leaves and tree branches, see the squirrels running and jumping from one tree to another, and birds searching for food and flying here and there. If you are surrounded by these things, then you are in nature and you can get all of its benefits.

Feminine Creativity

The Divine Feminine in all of us is associated with creative energy and life force energy, the feminine craves creativity.

It is not uncommon to feel stressed, anxious and down in the dumps from time to time, especially during times of hardship or transition. Thankfully, from simple doodling to singing your favorite song, moments of intentional creativity can come to the rescue, no matter your current lot in life.

When you find yourself stressed out, unwind by doing creative things you enjoy; painting, dancing, photography, sewing, cooking, decorating, crocheting, writing, gardening, entertaining guests. Expand your mind to see where in your life you are creating something out of nothing.

Being creative helps you become better problem solver in all areas of your life and work. Creativity helps you see things differently and better deal with uncertainty. Studies show that creative people are better able to live with uncertainty, entertain themselves and increase their control over emotional pain and depression.

Socializing over creative acts promotes more happiness; studies indicate it promotes better health too. So take advantage of the socializing benefits of creative acts and enjoy sharing and making new friends.

Pamper Your Divine Self

Let your body know it is safe. Let your body know you love her. Find ways you enjoy de-stressing and unwinding so your cave woman body is not fearful and feels safe enough to release excess stored energy (fat).

CHAPTER 2

The Divine Feminine Diet

A key component of divine feminine radiance is what type of food you're consuming. The fastest way to change your consciousness is through food.

The Divine Feminine Diet is the art of conscious selection of healthy foods based on the season, environment, hereditary issues, time of day, lifestyle, health disorder, etc.

The Divine Feminine Diet is based on the concept that the definition of "healthy food" is relative and varies from person to person. What is healthy for one may be unhealthy for another.

The Divine Feminine Diet is not just about what to eat, but also about "how to eat".

Whether it's shedding pounds, losing bloat, clearing up your skin, improving your digestion, or just gaining more energy, The Divine Feminine Diet will help remove any imbalances which may be preventing you from becoming the healthiest, most radiant and thriving version of your divine self.

The Magic of Mother Nature

You can't fool mother nature. Your body needs the real deal. Real, organic, fresh, fruits and vegetables that are home-prepared in a very simple way will have you shining from the inside out.

Mother Nature had a plan for healthy eating for our ancient ancestors that didn't involve refrigeration, preservatives or artificial ingredients. Instead, bread, beans, cheese, yogurt, butter, wild or shepherded meats, fish, fruit, olive oil, honey, and wine were the versatile, flavorful and beautifully rich foods we find mentioned in the ancient Bible.

In that refrigerator-less, non-industrialized promised land flowing with milk and honey, excess milk would have spontaneously soured and preserved itself and wheat grains magically fermented and changed into a healthy life sustaining food called bread. Since Mother Nature gave us the food and put beneficial organisms in the food in the first place, we must seriously consider this must have been the perfect eating plan.

Over Educated

We think we are so educated and advanced in our modern lifestyle but we have lost our common sense and ability to think for ourselves. We can't see the obvious staring us in the face; man and their science will never improve on Mother Nature. The Creator, created our bodies and created the earth with everything we need to live and thrive on. This has been working for hundreds of thousands of years but we have reached a point that man's interference with nature and the natural order of things has caused a decline in our health and the health of the planet.

Food Experts

There is no end to food experts, fad diets, diet books, celebrity diets, food rules and food pyramids. Believe me I know, I've read a few hundred of them myself. They claim to be based on science but that changes every few years, because it is the science of man, not Mother Nature. An example, the latest diet fads preach fruit fear. Any nutritionist, doctor or self proclaimed health expert who tells you to limit or not to eat fruit, nature's most perfect food, is out of touch with reality.

In the past science and "experts" told us not to eat fat and low-fat and non-fat was the rage, currently the keto diet is all the rage, saying fat is now good for you. We were told not to eat eggs, now they tell us that was wrong and eggs are a perfect food. Soy was good, then it was bad, now it is good again. They told us carbs were bad for us, now gluten is the big bad wolf.

The truth is, it isn't food that is the problem, it is what is being done to the food that is causing problems.

You don't have to understand science or depend on experts to tell you what to eat and what not to eat to take control of your health. You have the same body the cave woman had, evolution has not changed that. Just like our ancient ancestors, you need the real food that Mother Nature provides for you, as she always has from the beginning of time. The science of man is in its infancy, Mother Nature is supreme.

Dieting

If you are like most women you have been on many diets and may have developed an unhealthy relationship with food. You may fear anything you eat is going to make you fat or sick. You may obsess over labels and ingredients taking the joy out of eating and shopping for food. It has become such a chore to try to eat healthy you may even hate thinking about food and wish you didn't have to eat it, shop for it or prepare it.

In the U.S., nearly half of us are on a diet and two-thirds of us are overweight or obese. Clearly, the diets most Americans are using to try to peel off pounds don't work. Fad diets, gimmicky products, and celebrity diet plans are all part of the problem. One half of dieters quit within the first month of these unrealistic plans. My clinical experience is that compliance with any restrictive diet is almost zero!

A diet plan that banishes your favorite food forever is going to fail. We all have trigger points that will cause us to cave in to our appetites sooner or later and we will abandon the temporary weight loss diet.

Many studies now concur that dieting makes you fat. Studies have shown that teenagers who diet are statistically three times more likely to be fat in five years time.

Most people already know what they should and shouldn't eat, which foods cause them to gain weight and lose weight, which foods give them energy and which ones make them feel terrible. You don't need an experts opinion to tell you what you already know about your own body.

Nutrient dense foods such as fruits, vegetables, beans, nuts, seeds and whole grains are filling and healing. Choose a plan that works for your personality and lifestyle. Think about what did and didn't work the last time you were on a diet. Was it too restrictive? Didn't provide enough structure? Ask yourself: How long can I stay on this? If you can't stick with it in the long run, you'll be right back where you started after a couple of months.

Most weight loss diets require a lot of self control and will power, this is why they fail. You can take temptation and will power out of the equation by turning food choices into a habit, something you do automatically without having to think about it.

- In the evening decide what you are going to eat the following day and write it down.
- Go to the kitchen and make whatever preparations may be necessary to make it happen.
- If you work or go to school you may need to prepare and pack a lunch the night before so all you have to do is grab your bag and walk out the door.
- You may need to take something out of the freezer to thaw.
- You may want to cut up veggies to make your dinner preparation quicker when you get home the following evening.
- You may need to pick up something at the market if you are missing ingredients for your desired meals.

By preplanning your daily meals you eliminate temptations, you don't have to make any choices or decide what you are going to eat, it's already been decided and prepped. This will eliminate temptation to grab fast food or order pizza because you are hungry and can't think of anything good to eat or fast and easy to make.

Weight Loss

Weight loss is a bonus of the divine lifestyle, but the main draw is that you will feel amazing. And when you feel it inside, you will glow on the outside. Put health at the heart of everything and you will enjoy reaping the endless benefits. Given that eating fresh fruits and vegetables can help prevent and fight everything from diabetes to cancer, filling your body with them doesn't sound like such a bad idea.

Compare the standard American diet of toxic meat, hormone filled dairy and processed food full of sugar and fat, that belongs in a bin more than it does in the cupboards of your home, to a diet rich in life giving vitamin and minerals packed in natural goodness. It's easy to see why you will feel energized and satiated. If you are really serious about losing weight you need to be completely honest with yourself about what you are eating.

No calorie or carb counting or portion restriction is required when eating healthy and natural carbohydrates found in fruits and veggies which are vital for the brain, red blood cells and the nervous system. Diets high in complex carbohydrates not only help shed excess weight but prevents a range of chronic illnesses. Put more plants on your plate.

A study of high carb plant based diets found that body weight decreased in participants who ate lots of complex carbohydrates with no animal products or oil in sight. A plant based diet of fruits, vegetables, beans, nuts and seeds and whole grains are packed with fiber goodness, doing wonders for the digestive system and helping you feel full and satiated, preventing overeating.

Opposite of this is the popular low carb diets which don't differentiate complex carbs from real whole food, and simple carbs from unnatural processed frankinfood, causing confusion and keeping people from eating enough healthy real food. The diet works for a short time and you do lose weight initially because you are cutting out sugar and flour but the excess fat and meat diet when followed for more than a few months begins taking a toll on your health. Because it is not sustainable when you stop the low carb diet the lost weight come back on. There is more to health than the number on the scales.

Weight Loss Tips Aside From Food:

- Drink water and lots of it. This is the simplest and maybe the most effective thing you can do to aid fat loss. Good old H2O is the only way to go!
- Preplan tomorrow's meals, write it down and prepare tomorrow's lunch and bag it so it is ready to go. You are

creating a habit, no choices and no willpower required to keep on track.

- Eat slowly, put your fork down between bites and chew your food well.
- Not eating 4hours before you go to bed is a small lifestyle change that will make your weight loss efforts more effective. When you want a night time snack remind yourself that it only takes ten pounds to drop a dress size.
- If you shed just 1 pound, you'll take 4 pounds of pressure off of your knees. Drop 10 pounds and you'll take 40 pounds of pressure off.

Five Ways To Get Fat:

- Eat too little
- Eat too much
- Eat late at night
- Snacking
- Eating 3-5 times daily
- Chronic dieting; trains your body to be very efficient at storing fat. It can turn protein and carbohydrates into fat, resulting in no matter what you eat it winds up stored as fat.

Remember:

No diet that requires willpower, or deprivation or causes guilt is going to work.

You Must Create Your Own Divine Diet

Your Divine Feminine human body is a magical vessel holding your soul which is why it is called your Temple. Love it, nourish it, be kind to it and take care of it on your terms. This is your life, your body, your responsibility.

To think we should all be on the same "diet" and eat the same foods is ridiculous. We all have unique health challenges and nutritional requirements. We are different ages, live different lifestyles and have different activity levels. We have different cultural backgrounds and enjoy different foods. Therefore it only makes sense to create your own eating plan that suits your lifestyle and level of commitment. Not a diet that someone else made up and sets rules to and not just a temporary diet for weight loss or illness, but a healthy lifestyle you will follow for the rest of your life.

Your very own diet, made and designed by you and policed by you, is the very best chance you have to have the stamina to reshape your body and improve your health. Good health is much more than your weight. Plenty of people who look fit on the outside develop illnesses and have heart attacks. Being thin on the outside doesn't necessarily mean you are healthy on the inside.

No one likes to be labeled, put in a box or stereotyped. The same is true for a meal plan or lifestyle label. As soon as you make claim to a diet label you take on the rules and regulations of that diet, which causes you stress and feeling the need to live up to your claim for fear of being judged or scoffed at if you are caught "cheating" or feel guilty because you didn't stick to someone else's guidelines. I prefer to call my diet, mostly plant based, and other people can mind their own business.

When I say "diet" I am talking about daily, nutrient dense food choices, for all around good health. Your weight will work itself out once you are healthy enough. Your plan may be to lose weight but your body may have other ideas. Your intelligent body will use all nutrients and resources to heal the most life threatening conditions first and work its way to the least life threatening last. To your dismay your extra weight may be considered stored fuel the body thinks it may need to keep you alive as it is healing you, therefore it isn't interested in releasing your fat in a hurry.

If your weight loss is slow take comfort in knowing your body is healing things you probably don't even know are going wrong.

Often, with a few small changes to your daily activity, food choices, de-stressing and other habits, you can wind up losing weight steadily and overcoming health challenges once and for all. Your body will release stored fat when it isn't under threat and is healthy.

When you devise your own eating plan you will be more likely to stick with it.

- First listen to your Divine Feminine body
- Listen to your intuition
- Learn about ancient traditional food
- Use muscle testing or a pendulum to connect to your subconscious which knows everything going on inside your body. These tools will help you know which foods your body likes and will heal you and which ones are causing you problems.

Personal Food Preferences

Those who believe strongly that eating a raw plant-based diet will make them strong and healthy tend to have good results. Likewise those who fervently believe that eating organic whole foods, including meat and dairy in the tradition of their ancestors is the route to their optimal health also tend to have good results. If you believe a particular food will heal you, chances are that it will benefit your body, even if it sometimes goes against conventional wisdom. The most important thing is to eat a balanced diet full of nutrient dense foods which are vital to good health and a sense of well-being.

The foods you Do eat are more important to your health and

weight than the foods you Don't eat. This is the opposite of what modern diets tell you.

80/20 Rule

I personally find it very difficult to do most things 100% perfect all the time. This is where the 80/20 rule comes into play. If I can eat healthy, real foods 80% of the time, then I have 20% to relax, if need be.

Let me encourage you not to let your food rule your life. Yes, choose the best when possible, and certainly, don't use your 20% when buying food at the grocery store (sorry no cookies or sodas). The point is that you have 20% to play with when you need it and that makes life much more enjoyable and less stressful. Once your diet consists of 80% real, healthy food and 20% of the other, you can always up your healthy percentage and lower your unhealthy percentage.

If this is to vague or you need more structure and accountability the One Free Meal per Week plan may work better for you.

One Free Meal per Week

No one likes to feel denied, deprived, limited or live under rules. When you make a commitment to eat healthy you will have to cut out some not-so-good-for-you foods you may enjoy.

Once you create your own personal meal plan you are comfortable with and will commit to, allow yourself the freedom to eat whatever you want for one meal per week, without judgement or guilt. That is only 52 times a year which won't cause you harm but gives you a wicked meal to look forward to often enough to keep you eating healthy and on track the majority of the time.

Three Bite Rule

When you really want a desert or have a piece of birthday cake at the party or join in on the toast at a wedding celebration and you are sick and tired of always being the one on a diet, use the three bite rule; have three bites and no more. This way you can enjoy yourself and not feel deprived without totally polluting your body, you just have to be careful that you don't have too many special occasions! Life is a special occasion and some people celebrate everything, which is good, just don't do it with food all of the time.

The longer you eat real food, raise your vibration and clean your body out you will find the sweet food you once enjoyed will taste too sweet and you will not miss them or crave them. Frying oil will smell nauseating, other peoples food will begin to taste too salty and you actually begin to crave a salad. Best of all you wont feel deprived any more because you enjoy the real food you are eating, of your own choice, and you will love how good you look and feel.

Appetite

Eat for the body you want, not for the body you have. Reconfiguring your appetite is not an impossible task, it's a matter of replacing bad habits with good habits. Once you have made your personal investment in creating your own meal plan and have made progress in your health and weight you will without a doubt know how much better off you are, which helps you stay on track and eat less.

With a little regular fasting and increase in water your stomach will shrink to it's proper size, the size of your balled up fist, and your appetite will automatically decrease.

Hunger

When we are not suffering from starvation because of food shortage, we get hungry because we are lacking nutrients. When the body needs vitamins and minerals it makes you hungry to get you to eat and give it what it needs. When we eat processed non-foods, no matter how much we eat, whether we are fat or skinny, we are under-nourished and lacking in vital nutrients which makes us hungry and sometimes have ravenous appetites. As you improve your food choices and properly nourish your body your appetite, cravings and hunger will decrease.

Food Portions

Smaller plates lead to smaller portions, and since many people still find the need to clean their plate you can cut a significant amount of calories just by reducing your portions sizes between 20 and 30%. The smaller plates and bowls can also trick your brain into thinking that you are consuming more than you actually are. If you see that you have eaten a full plate of food, you are likely to think that you have eaten enough.

When your food presentation is brightly-colored, it triggers your brain to eat less. It can also make food that you may not be as enthusiastic about eating seem more appetizing. If you focus on eating a rainbow color of fruits and vegetables throughout the week, you also will likely get all the nutrients you need to maintain good health.

Food Addiction

Addictive food behavior, whether it's binge eating, comfort eating, eating the wrong kinds of food or just plain overeating, is not a life sentence. It's something that with a reasonable amount of work, information and support from those around you, can be overcome. But it is going to take love for your divine self and extreme self care to do it. Food addiction is a real thing, it's not your fault but must be understood and addressed if it is a problem for you.

Sugar and flour are white powders that are as addictive as cocaine and heroine. Just like cocaine and heroine come from plants, sugar and flour come from plants that are refined, highly processed, concentrated and ground into a fine white powder, which affect the addictive brain pathways in the same ways drugs of abuse do.

The food industry has taken wholesome plant foods and turned them into drugs of abuse and put sugar and flour in everything you like; bread, cake, pasta, soda, cookies, doughnuts, and pancakes to name just a few.

When you have strong food cravings or uncontrollable hunger or an insatiable appetite, your addictive brain pathways have been highjacked. You are now a junkie. No amount of self control will overcome the addiction, you have to stop eating the foods causing the addiction.

Just like you have to completely stop smoking or using cocaine or heroine to overcome the cravings and addiction, food is no different. You have to completely stop eating the offending foods, not mostly stop or even allow yourself a little treat now and then, because just like drugs, the cravings and addiction will come back overpowering your willpower and taking over your brain once you allow it back in your body.

When you are tempted to have just one little treat, you have to throw up a mantra and say "This is not my food. I don't eat this food." Just as a smoker has to have a mantra "I am not a smoker" when they have a craving to smoke.

This is one area you have to implement extreme self-care or you will never break your food addiction habits. No amount of information, education, logic, love, desire or diet plan can break addictions. The only way to overcome the addiction is to eliminate and stay away from the food “drugs”, which are flour and sugar, forever.

When you are creating your personal, healthy, divine diet for yourself take this information into consideration. If you have food addiction issues you can’t allow yourself the Three Bite Rule or the Weekly Free Meal, if it includes sugar or flour.

Some peoples brains are more addictive than others, sugar and flour plague us with varying degrees of cravings, however sugar and flour contribute to insulin and weight problems for all of us.

Truly you have to accept that food addiction is a real thing just like being addicted to anything, alcohol, cigarets, drugs, etc. and must be treated as such. You may want to consult a professional to help you in a way you resonate with, maybe releasing trapped emotions, professional counseling, hypnosis, a support group or a buddy or private trainer who makes you accountable. Or check yourself into a fasting or whole food retreat where your food or juices are prepared for you and you will get the support you need while you are going through withdrawals. Once you suffer through that you will never want to have to do it again.

When you love yourself, love your body and love your life enough you will seek out the help you need to make better choices. There is no shame in needing help. We all need help sometimes.

Cook at Home

Unless you cook and prepare your own food, you can’t control your diet, and you are giving control of the most important elements of your life to corporations that don’t care about your health. The best way to be healthy is to cook and prepare your own food as much as possible.

- Homemade meals, treats and snacks are always best.

- Organic and vegetarian restaurants are the next best choice.
- In a pinch health stores will have some decent organic fruits and snacks.

Menus and Shopping Lists

If you plan your meals in advance, you are more likely to choose healthy options when you go to the store with a list for your weekly shopping trip. Make sure that you get a variety of different foods in your diet. We tend to buy the same foods over and over again. Most people only eat about 20 different foods all of the time. Planning ahead can also reduce the temptation to get takeout or make poor meal choices such as fast food or frozen meals.

Eating small portions of delicious, beautifully prepared, well thought out meals is almost impossible without planning ahead.

- Make the time to make a weekly meal plan, to include smoothies, juices and snacks.
- Make a shopping list of all the ingredients needed for each meal.
- Go to your garden, farmer's market, health store, grocery store, etc.
- Prep the food, wash, chop, roast, bag and freeze to save time preparing the meals.

You should be able to make a good pant based meal and have it on the table within 30 minutes.

Holidays, Parties and Social Gatherings

Eating food with friends and family is a celebration of life and spirit. Don't pass up a good time or social gathering because of food. Eat a little before you go or take a beverage and a dish of yummy food you love and share it with others. If that isn't appropriate take some raw nuts to nibble on if you know there won't be much there you want to eat. It's better to be a little hungry than to pollute your body.

A goddess doesn't pass up a good time with good people over differences of food choices. If you plan ahead and it is appropriate you could use an upcoming social gathering as your one "free meal" for the week. Or you could apply the Three Bite Rule: take only three bites of the desert or birthday cake, and leave the rest, so that you can participate and join in the celebrations.

Your Goddess Body - Your Choice

Nowhere is there a rule written that you have to eat and drink what everyone else in the room is eating and drinking. You have a choice and you shouldn't be embarrassed to exercise it, in good taste, of course. Be polite but firm when passing on a food or drink that doesn't agree with you. You are a Divine Feminine, a Goddess, you do not cave into others desires or opinions about what a Goddess eats and drinks.

When You Are The Hostess

If you are hosting a dinner party you can lead by example and keep it simple but tasty. Such as wild salmon served with a spicy sauce, oven roasted tomatoes with garlic, a simple salad and sliced fresh fruit for dessert. Or you could throw an outdoor BBQ party with vegetarian fare such as black bean burgers, veggie shish-ka-bobs and grilled pineapple. Keep an elegant, oversized pitcher filled with spa water; ice, fruit, herbs and filtered water, to encourage guests to enjoy the healthy infused water alternative. Your soiree can be fun, divinely delicious and nourishing.

Traveling

Whether you are traveling by car or plane or camping, travel can be stressful especially when you aren't familiar with the stores and restaurants. Pack your own meals and snacks so you don't go hungry and are tempted to eat junk. A little organizing and preparation ahead of time will keep you on your Goddess path.

Divine Feminine Foods

Nutrition is not low fat. It's not low calorie. It's not being hungry and feeling deprived. It's nourishing your body with real, whole foods so that you are consistently satisfied and energized to live your divine life to the fullest.

Make food choices that honor your health and taste buds while making you feel well. You do not have to eat perfectly to be healthy. You will not suddenly get a nutrient deficiency or gain weight from one snack, one meal, or one day of eating. It's what you eat consistently over time that matters.

We don't have to live a primitive life, live off the grid, emulate the indigenous cultures or thumb our nose at modern culture to be more natural and healthy. We are contemporary women living in a modern world. If we do not have the time or the inclination to properly prepare and grow our own food then we must find cooks and bakers who can prepare it for us.

I support local biodiverse farming, raw milk, ethical meat production, real-food, traditional food preparation, nutrient dense diets, healthy fats and organic sustainable living, but that doesn't mean I have to be the cook, baker or farmer. That is the beauty of living in our modern age, we have options.

Grow your own organic fruits and vegetables and herbs for food and medicine if possible, if not then buy them locally from farmers and farmers markets, co-ops, or garden in a community garden space.

Our Creator had a plan for healthy eating that didn't involve refrigeration, preservatives or artificial ingredients. Learn to prepare meals using traditional methods, use raw food, raw honey, soaked grains, raw nuts and sprouted seeds.

Best Goddess Foods to Eat:

- Organic vegetables
- Organic greens and herbs
- Organic fruits
- Soaked legumes, nuts and seeds
- Sprouts
- Whole grains: amaranth, brown rice, buckwheat, polenta, millet, oats, quinoa, sorghum, teff, organic wheat (always soak grains)
- Super Foods: spirulina, chlorella, blue green algae, wheat grass, alfalfa, barley, kamut, nutritional yeast, bee pollen
- Raw nuts, nut butters, nut milks
- Coconut oil, coconut butter, unsweetened coconut flakes, coconut sugar
- Olive oil, avocados
- Vegetable broths and potassium broths
- Pasture raised organic meats, dairy and eggs, sparingly
- Wild fish, shellfish and fish roe
- Organic herbs and spices
- Unrefined salt, Himalayan salt
- Filtered or local spring water, not tap or bottled water
- Raw honey, local and manuca, maple syrup grade B, Stevia, Monkfruit

What Not To Eat

The following are low vibrational foods:

- Processed sugar
- White flour products
- Soda pop, energy drinks
- Margarine, vegetable oils, hydrogenated oils
- Deep fried food
- Factory-Farm raised meats, dairy, eggs and farm-raised fish

Foods to Avoid or Partake Sparingly:

- Animal products, use healthy plant substitutes when possible, not all processed substitutes are healthy as advertised
- Processed fruit juice, drink only freshly juiced fruit for a juice fast or a shot of dense nutrition

Following your own personal tailored dietary guidelines is not as difficult as it may seem, because for every food that is bad for you, there are plenty of alternative, beneficial and tasty foods.

Fresh Herbs Will Change Your Life

There is nothing quit like the delectable taste of fresh herbs. They are readily available and are easy to grow in gardens, flower beds, pots and inside the house. Fresh herbs have been used for cooking and medicinal purposes from the beginning of time. They are a cooks indispensable culinary friend and the maker of gourmet greatness on the plate.

Using lovely herbs, even the basic ones like parsley, thyme and rosemary add color, taste and visual appeal to a dish. Herbs can add brightness, life and a palate pleasing effect to your dishes.

I am lucky enough to have my own gardens full of many herbs; thyme, sage, oregano, rosemary, mint, lemon balm, lavender, savoy, basil, cilantro, dill, marjoram, tarragon, and more. Such availability is a dream come true for me.

Buying Herbs: Today it is easy to find fresh herbs at farmer's markets, supermarkets and ethnic markets. They may be boxed, tied in bundles or fresh in pots.

To keep herbs at their best remove any rubber bands and trim off the root ends and the lower parts of the stems to prevent the tops from wilting.

Wrap the trimmed but unwashed herb bunches in damp paper towels and put them in a heavy duty zip-lock bag filled with a little air, which cushions the herbs.

Store the herbs in the warmest part of the refrigerator, which is often the top shelf. Check the herbs daily using those that are the least perky and discarding any that have begun to spoil.

Wash Herbs Only When You Are Ready to Use Them: Excess moisture shortens their life in the refrigerator. If I can get away without washing them at all I do. When they are from my organic garden I don't wash them.

To wash herbs, put them in a large bowl of cool water and swish them around to release any sand or grit. Lift the herbs out of the water and spin them dry in a salad spinner or gently blot them dry with a paper towel or roll them in a clean dish towel.

Cutting Herbs: A sharp knife is imperative for chopping herbs. A dull knife will crush and bruise the tender leaves giving you a blackened look rather than green. I use scissors to cut a small amount of herbs or chives whose stringy fibers make it difficult to get a clean cut with a knife.

You can save leftover chopped herbs for a day or so but they become highly perishable once chopped.

Fresh Herbs: There is one golden rule for fresh herbs; always add them toward end of cooking to keep their delicate flavor and color.

Use the whole herb. When a recipe calls for only one part of the herb, such as the leaves, reserve the remaining parts for other uses. Tender stems can be tied with twine and used in soups and stocks. Woody stems can go to the grill like fragrant wood chips. Herb blossoms in season can be added to salads and pastas as a garish.

Over Abundance: If you have too large a crop or purchased more than you can use or they have passed their prime, there are a lot of things you can do with them. Adding them to vinegars, oils, butter, making them into paste or pesto or preserving them in ice cube trays with olive oil or dehydrating them, ensures none goes to waste.

Dried Herbs: When color counts dried herbs are a poor substitute for fresh. Dried herbs are best used when the dish is very wet, like a sauce when the herbs have time to reconstitute in the liquid.

When substituting dry herbs for fresh herbs in a recipe, use only 1/3 the amount called for fresh herbs because of their condensed flavor.

Stocking Your Kitchen

True health care reform starts in the kitchen. The ingredients you stock up on will vary depending on your culture, if you choose to eat meat, plant based, vegetarian, vegan or mostly raw.

Refrigerated Items:

- Fruits
- Vegetables
- Salad greens
- Mushrooms

- Herbs
- Sprouts
- Butter, ghee
- Eggs
- Nuts
- Nut milk
- Nut butter
- Meat

Pantry Items:

- Unsweetened coconut flakes
- Chia seeds
- Flax seeds
- Oats
- Raw cocoa
- Sprout seeds
- Coconut oil
- Olive oil
- Organic spices
- Real salt, Himalayan salt
- Nut butters
- Herbal teas
- Beans, legumes, lentils
- Quinoa, polenta, etc.

Freezer Items:

- Organic fruits and vegetables
- Organic meat
- Peeled and halved bananas for smoothies
- Raw nuts, to keep from going rancid
- Wild blueberries

Kitchen Tools and Equipment

- VitaMix or high powered blender
- Juicer
- Colander
- Cutting board
- Chef's knife
- Paring knife
- Tea kettle
- Baking sheet
- Spatula
- Tongs
- Whisk
- Veggie peeler
- Grater
- Kitchen shears
- Spiralizer
- Garlic press
- Zester
- Steamer basket
- Nut milk bags
- Sprouting sack, jar or containers
- Glass storage containers
- Parchment paper
- Stainless Steel pans #18-10 (not #18-08, they are thinner and warp)

Having the proper kitchen tools will enable you to make delicious and beautiful food. Learn to cut, chop, slice, dice, grate, julienne, spiralize, juice, shred and puree your vegetables and fruits. It is amazing how the flavors change and the beautiful presentation is much more appetizing.

Imagine what our ancient foremothers could do with food if they had all of the tools and appliances we have in our kitchens today!

Creating Your Own Diet

If you think I did not create a specific enough outline for you to follow for the Divine Feminine Diet, it is by design. In the following chapters you will learn how your body works, what it needs for nourishment, and encourage you to trust your inner knowing and intuition. You will be empowered to make good choices for your own well-being depending on your lifestyle and level of commitment. Part of being a Divine Feminine is being empowered and confident to make your own choices and create your own experiences. Remember it's effort and progress not perfection that will transform your health.

Part of the experience of having a mortal body is to learn to control your mind and body rather than let them control you. In addition, you didn't come to earth just to be one of the masses to be controlled by religions, governments, big business and "experts", which all rule with fear causing you to doubt your own power and divinity.

You came to earth at this time to take on human form and bring with you gifts from another world into this one. You came armed with knowledge, training and the tools you need to navigate earth's training ground to expand your soul.

We each have the power to discover our own answers, which will always point us to our highest well-being, to live our best life as individuals.

You have the ability and responsibility to be in control of your health and well-being and it is not as complicated as modern society would have us believe. Creating a healthy Divine Feminine diet and lifestyle is well within your reach. You have the spiritual tools of intuition, prayer, meditation, personal revelation and help from your ancestors and spiritual family beyond the veil, to help you know what choices are in your best interest.

CHAPTER 3

Eat Real Food From Mother Earth

> ***"Healthy eating isn't about counting fat grams, dieting, cleanses, and antioxidants; Its about eating food untouched from the way we find it in nature in a balanced way; Whole foods give us all that we need to perfectly nourish ourselves." Pooja Mottl, Natrual Foods Chef***

If a grocery store has a "health food" section, what does that make the rest of the store? 80% of the supermarkets food sections are all processed foods, frozen, dry or canned including snacks, "healthy" bars, cereals, processed meats, junk food, most salad dressings, sauces, sweets, ice-cream, candy and chewing gums are unhealthy items disguised as food.

Your Divine Feminine body deserves the best. Stop paying for food that doesn't serve you and invest in nutrition that your body craves and deserves. Eating well is a form of self-respect and self-love.

Clean Eating is a phrase that we hear a lot these days, but what does it really mean? Simply put, clean eating refers to a diet made of organic, whole, unprocessed ingredients. Most processed foods like frozen dinners and "from-the-box" meals contain hidden sugars, unhealthy fats, refined grains, and empty calories. Focusing on clean, plant predominant, whole foods in their most natural state instead, will provide your body with vital nutrients and fewer calories.

It's time to return back to eating the way we did before the food industry ruined food. Every time you eat or drink, you are either feeding disease or fighting it.

We are living today because our ancestors survived eating off of the land, as nature intended it to be. Today we are sick and dying of man made diseases because of the fake food we eat. This is the first time in history our children will not live as long as their parents will and it is all because of their diets.

You are a living being and you need living food to feed the cells of your body. If you eat dead food you are going to feel dead and die sooner. Death brings death. Eat to live, don't eat just for taste. Your cells are continually renewed and you always have a chance to recreate yourself.

Our health problems are stemming from the fact that we aren't eating real food anymore, we are eating food-like products. Don't eat anything that is incapable of rotting. The longer the "foods" shelf life is, the shorter your life will be. Dead foods are mucus and acid forming. They have no elements needed for digestion.

"Low-Fat" and "Sugar-Free" are usually code words for chemically laden, overly processed and unnatural. When you eat real food without labels it actually contains messages that communicate with every cell of the body. Good nutrition will prevent 95% of all diseases.

We spend trillions of dollars treating diseases, when we could be preventing the diseases by simply changing our diet.

Eating for Regenerative Health

Your body already knows how to heal itself. You are an angel who has come to earth to take on human form to be here in the dimension of slowed down time and space, to live within your own creation, see the results of your thoughts, actions and consciousness, to expand your soul. You brought all the tools you need with you. You are so much more than you think you are and have more power than you can imagine.

Do you love yourself enough to believe in yourself and allow yourself to change, without relying on someone or something else? If you want to heal it's simply about making the choice to let your body heal. Your body will cleanse itself, re- balance itself and detoxify itself. Get into attunement with your body rather than reaching out to the next new therapy or potion that comes along, hoping that will be the next new thing that heals you.

All you have to do is remember who you are, believe in yourself, give your body what it needs and take away what is harming it, and make the choice to let your body heal.

There has always been disease and illness on earth but we are enjoying life on earth today because our ancient ancestors survived by living off of the land and out in nature. They ate real food, organic, fresh, whole food with the seasons and drank clean water. We suffer from obesity and man-made degenerative illnesses because of the way we eat and drink today.

Your Diet Should Change With the Seasons and Your Age

One's diet should change with the seasons and with the place they live in. The primary reason why people fall sick when seasons change is that we continue doing the same thing, eating the same foods day after day. We are heedless to the gentle prodding of nature which suggests we change our habits with the seasons.

You must adapt yourself and your lifestyle to remain in sync with nature for optimal health through all seasons.

Not only that, our diet continues to be the same year after year even as we grow older. The child, adolescent, adult and seniors in the house eat the same food. This is inappropriate. Every age group has its own nutritional needs which have to be met.

During childhood our digestive ability is at its peak. Hence rich nutritional diet consumed will be optimally digested, the nutrients will be saved in the body and the reserves used for several years to come.

The adolescent also has a fairly strong constitution or digestive ability and needs nutrients particularly to nourish the brain and nervous system to deal with the stress and intellectual demands of modern day education.

As it ages the body needs more frequent maintenance and rejuvenation in order to keep it functioning optimally. As the human body grows older, tissue regeneration and metabolism slows down. your physique loses considerably of its natural ability to burn calories quickly. Over the age of 40 the body has lesser capacity to absorb and assimilate nutrients from the food consumed. All this can manifest into an older looking body, hormone imbalance, lack of interest in life, depression and diminished libido. A carefully designed diet is required by the body to battle the deterioration of the tissue.

In senior years with the downward trend of the body's functions, the diet has to be modified accordingly to provide the right nutrition while causing minimal strain on the organs.

Women expend 75-150 fewer calories per day each decade from their 30s until age 70, leading to about a 20 per cent decline in muscle mass. Our activity drops away as we get older, particularly our vigorous activity and our resistance training, so our muscle mass tends to drop and the body no longer has enough fat-burning muscle reserves to keep up with the same amount of food it once could. However, consuming fewer calories every decade means there's a good chance of avoiding excess weight gain around the waist and reducing the associated risk of chronic disease in the process.

It's harder to stay lean as you get older, but gradually reducing portion sizes each decade can help to ward off the middle-age spread. As you get older discretionary food items really need to be tightened because your nutrient requirements don't decrease as you get older and you have to get those nutrients in less food.

Your eating plan should include:

- Eating mindfully
- Eat at least 80% healthy food
- Drink plenty of clean water
- Move your body
- Pay attention to how you feel after you eat
- Only eat food that makes you feel good and gives you energy
- Stop eating food that tastes good but makes you feel lousy
- Enjoy your food immensely but don't over eat
- Don't use food as a reward or eat for comfort or out of boredom or late at night
- Don't starve or binge or purge
- Don't diet or exercise to punish your body, but rather because you love and appreciate your Divine Feminine body and want to treat it well and keep it healthy so you can have an active, happy, long life.

Eating Organic Isn't a Trend, it is a Return to Tradition

It is important to eat pure, organic unadulterated foods that are right for you, in order to achieve optimal health, energy and happiness.

If you want foods as per your convenience, to suit your whims and eating urges, they are available at the supermarket 24/7. But those products available off the shelf at the supermarket, found neatly packaged and preserved for year round consumption, are NOT really organic. They are beautifully packaged and preserved dead bodies of things once living. It would be wrong to call them "organic". These mass-produced items are stripped of a major portion of their nutritive value during processing and also laced with preservatives and artificial colors and flavors for mass appeal.

It is not enough to merely purchase products marked "organic" at the grocery store. The food industry is catching on to the public's desire for organic food so they are making their refined processed food with organic ingredients. This is a sham, it is not healthy food even if it doesn't have added chemicals.

Organic food habits have to be coupled with making your lifestyle, your behavior and your mindset organic. The organic mindset is flexible. An organic lifestyle is to live in sync with nature, the changes in season, climatic conditions, availability of food products, etc. In order to adopt a truly organic, natural lifestyle it is important to be flexible and to adapt to nature. Re-wild yourself!

Five Reasons to Make the Organic Switch:

1. Certified organic farmers are held to a higher standard: Before a farm is eligible to receive the certified organic seal, a farm must document and practice organic farming practices for at least three years. Once certified, organic

farmers must reapply every year and undergo a strict annual inspection. The inspection is performed by a third party inspector. The farmers must be able to answer for their farming practices and provide documentation from seed to harvest. The inspector also conducts a plant and soil test on the farm. The requirements for organic farmers are consistent across the board, so all organic farmers must meet the same requirements and undergo the same annual inspection.

2. Certified organic produce is worth the price: Certified organic farmers pay big dollars to the government for their certification. Yes, it's sad that farmers growing the natural way must pay for a stamp of approval, but it's the current state of our nation and the food system. Not only do farmers pay for certification, which means lots of extra work through organic farming techniques and documentation, they also use natural, sometimes more costly, practices.

   Organic farmers may produce less strawberries and cucumbers, for example, due to exposure to natural conditions which synthetic pesticides and herbicides fight against. Sometimes this means losing 20% of the crop.

   Next time you see the package of $5 organic strawberries next to the $3 conventional berries, know the difference from seed to harvest is remarkably different; as well as the extra cost the farmer paid to guarantee the berries were grown as nature intended in unpolluted soil, using untreated seeds, utilizing natural pest control and fertilizers.

3. Buying certified organic allows you to vote with your dollar: It's easy to complain about toxic fertilizers and pesticides being used on our food supply, but complaining is not going to create much change. Companies understand one important currency: money. By purchasing organic

you're casting a vote. A vote for sustainable and natural practices that don't deplete the soil or leave synthetic toxins in our food.

By supporting local organic farms, you're putting money back into local people and your community, instead of big profit-driven companies. It's as easy as waking early on a Saturday morning and visiting a local farmer's market or finding the organic produce section in your local store.

Companies will never pay attention to the complaints if we don't start putting our money and talk together.

4. Certified organic is better for the body and environment: Certified organic farmers have a list which details the pesticides they may use on their organic farms. The pesticides must come from natural sources and include: soaps, fish emulsion, diatomaceous earth, neem, and more.

   Conventional farming practices regularly include spraying synthetic, opposite of natural, pesticides and herbicides which pollute the water, air, and food. Studies have shown an increased risk of cancer when rats are exposed to many of the toxins used on conventional farms. Around half of the synthetic chemicals used today are known to be carcinogenic.

   According to Unraveling GMOs: What They Are, How to Avoid Them, and How to Make a Difference, "By USDA requirements under the USDA Certified Organic Seal, farmers are not allowed to use synthetic pesticides, bio-engineered genes (GMOs), petroleum based fertilizers, and sewage sludge-based fertilizers. Why would anyone want to use those methods any way! Buying organic means saying "yes" to a cleaner environment and healthier bodies.

5. Certified organic means saying "NO" to GMO's. Today, consumers must worry about both carcinogenic pesticides and herbicides, and GMO's. GMO's are organisms whose

genes have been altered in a lab. So, while that papaya may look like a papaya, its genes are anything but a good ol' papaya. Fortunately, certified organic farmers must prove from seed to harvest that they don't use GMO seeds or plants. Unfortunately, when buying conventional produce there really isn't any sign, label, or disclaimer of an impostor.

Eat Less Meat, More Whole Foods and Mostly Plants

Most of us don't have the time, ability or resources to grow and cook all of our own food filled with love and energy, that we'd ideally want to ingest and feed to our family and friends. The following guidelines will help us get as close as we can in our modern world.

- Buy local when possible, organic, fresh or frozen, not canned.
- Eat some raw living food every day, if your digestive health allows it.
- The Mediterranean, Flexatarian and Plant Based Diets are good guidelines if you choose to eat meat or dairy. Simply limiting meat intake in favor of more plant foods all qualify as plant-based diets. Plant-based doesn't mean vegetarian or vegan unless you want it to.
- Eat more plants and less meat. The phytochemicals, antioxidants, and fiber, all of the healthful components of plant foods, originate in plants, not animals. If they are present, it is because the animal ate plants. So why should we go through an animal to get the benefits of the plants themselves? Your body has to use a lot of energy to break

down animal protein to extract the amino acids that came from plants in the first place.

Eat High Vibrational Energy Foods

High vibrational foods are typically in their purest form and connected to the earth. An organic apple directly off the tree is going to have a higher vibration than, for instance, the ones that are already cut up in a bag with some preservatives on them.

Foods shipped long distances lose their vibrational value because they didn't have a chance to ripen with the energy of the sun to maximize their vibrational quality. Choose local whenever possible for better food and to support your local farmers.

The sun is the key to everything as it infuses every plant with the energy to grow and reach their maximum health benefit. So, when choosing foods, think about how much direct sunlight they received. The packaged foods that are picked early, stored and shipped a long distance, receive way less time basking in the sunlight.

High vibration foods get their name because they provide energy and therefore raise the body's level to a higher frequency. They have the nutrients necessary to fuel the electrical currents in your body. These foods are natural and toxin-free. In general, high-vibration foods don't have chemicals, additives, or flavorings.

Any food consumed in its pure form gives off high energy, which your body absorbs when you eat it. Physically, your body responds to a higher vibration with increased blood flow to tissues, muscles and organs. Oxygen is carried in your blood and to the various systems throughout your body, nourishing it more optimally.

Within your body, your organs, muscles, cells and nerves all have a healthy level of vibration. When your body becomes out of balance, disease occurs.

Eat 5-13 Servings of Fruits and Vegetables Daily

One serving of fruit or vegetables equals half a cup, or about the amount you could hold in a cupped hand. Nutrition experts used to recommend five servings of fruits and vegetables per day, but that's probably not enough, according to the Centers for Disease Control and Prevention (CDC). Individual needs are different, depending on age, gender, and level of physical activity, you'll require between 5 and 13 servings of fruits and vegetables each day.

Eating plenty of fruits and vegetables is especially important, because the nutrients and fiber in these foods can help reduce high blood pressure, lower your risk of heart disease, stroke, and certain cancers, stave off eye and digestive problems, help the kidneys remove excess acid from the body and excrete it in urine and simply satisfy your hunger.

Tips for Beginners to Eat More Fruits and Vegetables

- Display your produce. Put your fruits and vegetables out on the counter or in a prominent position in the refrigerator, so that you'll be more likely to eat them.
- Cook vegetarian at least once every week, skip the meat and try a new vegetarian recipe for dinner. Increase it to 2 weekly meals, then 3 and so on, until you are eating a mostly plant predominant diet.
- Add fruits and vegetables to your favorite dishes. Find ways to incorporate fruits and vegetables into foods you already eat. For example, stuff your omelet with extra vegetables or pack your sandwich with veggies. Eat a veggie loaded salad every day, make a fruit or savory smoothie everyday.

Fruit Fear

When I was studying nutrition 20 years ago we were taught that sugar is bad and sugar is sugar no matter where it comes from, including fruit. Wrong! Most all weight loss diets will tell you to severely limit or omit fruit from your diet. Bad advise.

Eating whole fruit is loaded with fiber, water, minerals and significant chewing resistance, plus it is incredibly filling and easy to digest when chewed well. Fruit is juicy deliciousness, it's like a gift from the Goddesses. Fruit is the original fast food.

Science Lesson

Are you aware that there is such a thing as Sugar Spin? And according to how the sugar molecules spin, it will affect your health drastically? Right-Spin sugar molecules contribute to weight gain, diabetes and feeding cancer cells. While Left-Spin sugar molecules help you lose weight and gets a free ride out of your system. Human digestive enzymes have evolved to act upon Right-Spin sugar molecules, while often allowing Left-Spin forms to pass directly through.

You can find the harmful Right-Spin sugar molecules in all sugars concocted by Man in a laboratory, to include GMO fruits. Examples are white sugar, refined sugar, synthetic sugar, aspartame, and high fructose corn syrup. All of which are really just poison to your body. They taste good but they are still toxic to your body, cause inflammation and weaken your immune system. These include all products made with these sugars; sodas, sweetened beverages, cakes, candy, doughnuts, etc.

You can find the good Left-Spin sugars in Nature; honey, maple syrup, molasses, the sugars in non-GMO fruits, non-GMO coconut, to mention a few. Left-Spin sugars are good for you. Not only do they strengthen your immune system, they are also nutrient-rich.

Left-Spin sugars are quickly metabolized by the body and thus puts no extra load on the kidneys. Lab officials say, it doesn't appear to create fat, as most sugars do, possibly because of the rate at which it metabolizes.

Back to the Fruit

Fresh raw fruit is one of the most perfect foods on earth. It is full of electricity, sunshine and nutritious water which is full of vitamins, minerals, essential sugars and antioxidants.

Fruit is full of fiber, the exact kind and amount to slowly digest the sugars naturally found in each particular fruit. We have been trained to think of fruit as a snack, desert or treat, when in fact fruit is a real food with nutritional sustenance that can be a meal unto itself. A really good fruit cannot be improved, because Mother Nature has already done that.

The most wonderful thing about fruit is the simplicity of it. Imagine a sweet strawberry or watermelon or juicy mango or peach. Take a bite of it and taste the explosion of flavors in a ripe, high quality fruit. Sip it's luscious juice and chew it's soft flesh. There is no water more pure or alive than found in fresh fruit.

Add more ripe organic fruit to your diet. Our ancient ancestors picked them ripe off of the trees and vines and ate them all summer long and so should you.

Sugar

Your body does need carbohydrates, which are broken down into sugar in your body. This sugar is essential for your body to create energy to survive. A diet with adequate complex carbohydrates (from foods such as whole grains and legumes) as well as foods containing natural sugar (such as fruit) will fulfill this role.

However, it is not necessary to include processed sugary foods or added sugars in the diet in order for your body to make energy. The table sugars and high fructose corn syrup added during food processing and preparation, called added sugars, are viewed as a detriment to a healthy diet.

Fructose is fruit sugar and can cause harm when isolated and consumed in excess. However, there is not enough fructose in fresh fruit to cause concern.

Super Foods

This widely used term refers to foods that are chock full of nutrients. These foods include nuts, lacto-fermented vegetables, spirulina, blue-green algae, chlorella, wheat grass, alfalfa, barley, kamut, nutritional yeast, and bee pollen.

Raw Food

Foods in their pure state retain their nutrients and give off a higher vibration than if you cook them. Uncooked foods have the propensity to control allergic, digestive, and metabolic problems.

Raw food picked off the bushes, trees and vines are full of nutrient dense water, fiber, energy and enzymes to help digest the food. The more raw food you can add to your diet the better. Salads and green blender drinks are a great way to eat more vegetables and greens.

Fresh fruit is packed with goodness and should be eaten every day. Stuff yourself with raw fruits and vegetables as much as you can. Cooked and frozen are great too but will lack the enzymes to help digest them.

A quick note about vegetables; if you are experiencing digestive symptoms you may do better with cooked vegetables than raw, until you are healthier. Serious digestive damage can be made worse by raw vegetables that may be hard to digest, so choose soup over salads.

When a person has digestive or dental problems, to include young children and older folks, it is easier for them to chew and digest cooked food than raw food. Theoretically, no matter how healthy raw food may be, it becomes very unhealthy if it cannot be digested properly.

Grains, Nuts and Seeds

Grains, nuts and seeds are potentially new plants and trees packed full of fiber and nutrition. There are protections in grains that keep them from growing until conditions are perfect. Grains and seeds contain phytates and other substances designed to keep the grain from deteriorating until optimal conditions for germination to create new plants and trees. This is good for the seed but a bad thing for the human digestive tract. Soaking is a way that phytic acid can be broken down so that our bodies are able to have full access to the nutrients found in grains.

Most grains, nuts, seeds, and legumes contain phytic acid, which has been shown to block mineral uptake. Breaking down the phytic acid in these foods requires you to either soak, ferment, or sprout them before consuming, just as our ancient ancestors did.

Digestion: Grains that are barely on their way to becoming a new plant are easier to digest. It makes sense considering that the toughness is being broken down in favor of a new, tender plant.

Nutrients: Catching a plant at this stage means catching all the nutrients necessary for growth, the process makes those nutrients more accessible for our bodies. Another important factor is that there are many nutrients that aren't available in grains until they germinate, an important one is vitamin C.

Soaking: Our ancestors, and virtually all pre-industrialized peoples, soaked or fermented their grains before making them into porridge, breads, cakes and casseroles. Through scientific research, we are now able to understand why and how it all works.

Grains can be soaked in water or mixed with things like salt or something acidic like yogurt, whey or lemon juice.

Sprouting: Besides neutralizing various inhibitors, sprouting also increases the digestibility of nuts, seeds, grains, and legumes because soaking helps convert vegetable protein into simple amino acids. Complex carbohydrates will also break down into simpler glucose molecules. This is why you always want to soak your beans.

The sprouting of seeds is a fascinating natural phenomenon. In un-sprouted seeds, their enzymes are dormant and inhibited. However, when seeds are soaked and allowed to germinate and sprout, an incredible amount of enzymes are released. Enzymes are found in raw foods and are the spark of life! They are proteins that are needed for all the metabolic processes in your body to occur. The sprouting of seeds also releases wonderful vitamins, especially vitamin C and the spectrum of B vitamins. The seed transforms into something brand new, which has released much of its energy, but is much richer in nutrients. They're so very good for your health!

Before we had fire, we knew the value of sprouting grains, legumes and seeds. We knew instinctively that Nature had created them as potent nutritional bundles of health and energy. Without science at our disposal to tell us what we needed, we automatically germinated and sprouted these concentrated natural sources of vitamins, minerals, enzymes and amino acids. We built our bodies on them.

Salt

Himalayan Crystal Salt, Real Salt or Pink Salt, which comes from the depths of the Earth, are pristine because their minerals suspend in a crystalline structure, as a colloid. The colloidal form makes it easy for the body to absorb. Because it contains a lot of nutrients, they give off a high vibration.

Sea salt once was a good choice but because of the pollution in the oceans today the salt may be contaminated and contain plastic particles.

Processed table salt isolates sodium and removes the other minerals which is what causes water retention and high blood pressure. One more example of man interfering with nature and ruining a good thing. However table salt has iodine added to it because it was the easiest way to get it into the diets of people who didn't live by the ocean or eat seafood. Kelp salt is a good seasoning to have in your kitchen. Eat seaweed, seafood or take an iodine supplement if needed.

Chocolate

The mere mention of the word chocolate perks up most anyone. However, we aren't discussing chocolate as we know it, with added sugar, fat and wax. Instead, it's the raw form of chocolate, cacao, that should interest us. It has over 1,200 phytonutrients, vitamins, and minerals. All derivatives of it, such as cocoa butter, powder, and nibs are all healthy, delicious and efficient at raising your vibrational energy.

Oil and Seasonings

Fat and oil are easy fuels for the body to use as energy and it will always choose to use fat in your diet before it converts its own fat into energy. If you want to lose weight keep in mind added fat and oil are extra calories, with no nutritional value which you have to burn through before burning off any of your reserved energy (fat).

Good Fats and Flavorings:

- Coconut Oil is high in fatty acids, has analgesic, antifungal, and antiviral properties. It also contains lauric acid, which boosts metabolism.
- Extra Virgin Olive Oil
- Organic butter, Ghee
- Fresh Herbs
- Fresh Lemon
- Raw Apple Cider Vinegar
- Nutritional Yeast (tastes cheesy and a good source of vegetable protein)

Protein

No matter what diet you follow, whether you eat meat or not, protein is an essential part of a healthy diet. Along with carbohydrates, fats, water, vitamins and minerals, proteins are one of the 6 groups of essential nutrients for the human body.

Each protein is made up of a combination of up to 25 different amino acids, each serving its own purpose. There are 8 essential amino acids, meaning the body can't make them and they have to come from a food source (histidine, isoleucine, leucine, lysine, methionine, phenylalanine, threonine, tryptophan, and valine). From these, the other 17 amino acids can be made by the body.

Leafy greens have a considerable amount of protein and should be eaten daily. Greens have sufficient protein to build muscle in grazing animals. A variety of greens can supply all the protein we need to sustain each of our unique bodies.

Amino acids and proteins are the building blocks of life. When proteins are digested or broken down, amino acids are left. The human body uses amino acids to make its own proteins as needed to help the body:

- Break down food
- Grow
- Repair body tissue
- Perform many other body functions

When you consume animal protein, it is broken down in the gut to its amino acid or peptide components, before being transported in the blood to where they are needed.

This means when you eat meat, your body has to break the meat down to extract the amino acids. Protein does not stay protein. Your digestive system breaks down everything you eat into individual components to use as needed. This requires a lot of energy and work for your body. It is easier on your system to eat plant food with amino acids ready to use, which is where the animal got the amino acids in the first place.

We have been brain washed to believe we have to eat meat to get enough protein. This is a lie. Think about this; does the cow eat another cow to get it's protein? No. The cow eats grasses and plants which have the amino acids it needs to make it's own protein. We humans, gorillas and ox are the same. Eat more plants.

When the meat industry tried to feed cows meat and body parts of other cows to save money, they created mad cow disease.

Plant Protein

Plant protein is considered incomplete but preferred over animal protein. Being incomplete means that you need to eat a variety in order to obtain all 8 essential amino acids. Some of the most complete plant protein sources are quinoa, buckwheat, chickpea (garbanzo bean), pumpkin seed, nutritional yeast, spirulina, chlorella, soy beans, hemp seeds, chia seeds. A plants amino acid make up is only incomplete if that is the only plant you ever ate, and no others.

Plant Protein provides secondary benefits: Unlike animal protein, plant-based protein sources like beans, nuts, seeds, and dark leafy greens come with the added benefit of fiber and anti-inflammatory health benefits. It's ok to get protein from animal sources as well, if it's in your comfort zone, so long as quality is kept in mind. Animal proteins should be organic and grass-fed when possible and always eaten sparingly.

Protein is essential for health. We need to make sure we are getting enough to support cell repair, muscle growth, hormone health, and immune function. The good news is that it's easy. The key is to focus on high-quality protein sources. Focus on getting most of your protein from plants, balanced with quality animal-based protein, should you choose to incorporate it in your diet.

It's all about balance, and a well-balanced diet is not only key to optimal protein balance, but it's essential for optimal health as well.

Strong As An Ox

Patrik Baboumian is a strongman competitor and vegan, he is said to be the strongest man in the world. In the documentary *Game Changers* he says "If you want to be as strong as an ox you have to eat like an ox. Have you ever seen an ox eat meat?"

Animal Protein

Animal products such as beef, pork, lamb, poultry, fish, shellfish, milk and cheese though high in protein, are also high in saturated fats and cooked protein is harder to assimilate. Moreover, modern farming methods leave much to be desired in the quality of the meat that is full of antibiotics, growth hormones and pesticides.

Some weight loss programs recommend very high protein

diets of up to 200 grams of protein a day. This is way too high and long term can be dangerous for health.

- Protein breakdown creates side-products that give extra work to the kidneys and liver. If your kidneys are healthy and protein intake moderate, then this poses no problem. But if you have even mild kidney trouble and eat large quantities of protein, especially from meat, this will stress your kidneys and worsen your condition.
- Meat protein is acid-forming in the body, creating an ideal environment for bacteria to breed and diseases to take hold. Calcium (an alkalizing agent) is required to neutralize the pH in the blood, which can cause calcium imbalance and increase the risk of bone loss.
- Marked acid load to the kidneys also increases the risk for kidney stone formation.
- Though animal proteins are considered a complete protein source, they cause the blood to be acidic and thicken. Furthermore, some animal proteins are destroyed during cooking, rendering them less bioavailable to the body and may become "waste" that remains in the body, causing health issues.

Eat Meat Sparingly

"We cut the throat of a calf and hang it up by the heels to bleed to death so that our veal cutlet may be white; we nail geese to a board and cram them with food because we like the taste of liver disease; we tear birds to pieces to decorate our women's hats; we mutilate domestic animals for no reason at all except to follow an instinctively cruel fashion; and we connive at the most abominable tortures in the hope of discovering

some magical cure for our own diseases by them."
George Bernard Shaw, Man and Superman

Even though "humanely raised" can mean different things, it should never mean that:

- Animals are raised in cages
- Animals are raised in tightly crowded barns
- Animals aren't allowed to express their natural behaviors
- Animals are bred in ways that cause physical deformations
- Animals are routinely given food that risks making them sick

Unfortunately, most animals raised for meat, eggs, and dairy in America are raised in these ways. This is not healthy for the animals or for you as the consumer. Change will only happen as more people choose alternative products:

- Grass-fed
- Pasture raised, free range
- No antibiotics or hormones
- Processed (slaughtered) humanely

If Slaughter Houses Had Glass Walls

"If slaughterhouses had glass walls,
the whole world would be vegetarian."
Linda McCartney, Artist/Musician

We have the freedom to make choices but we also have to live with the consequences of those choices. When it comes to factory farming animals in inhumane conditions just so we have daily, affordable, tender meat on our plates, it is an abomination no matter how one tries to rationalize it. The majority of meat and animal products sold in grocery stores come from these conditions.

There are privately owned rural ranches that do a better job with their animals, but it is still a business and they are paid by the pound for each animal which takes precedence in their choices of care. There are a few small organizations that raise free range, grass fed, organic animals without hormones and antibiotics. They try to give the animals a happy, well cared for life right up to the day they are humanely killed for food.

Every living creature wants to live and fears pain and death. Animals have emotions and experience joy, fear and sadness. They are living sentient beings and should be treated as such. The ancients knew this and treated all living things with respect and gratitude when they took a life for their life.

Black Bean Burgers

My family loves these burgers. This is a great recipe to cut out or cut down your consumption of meat.

Ingredients:

- 1 ½ cups black beans
- 1 cup short grain brown rice
- 1 cup walnuts, roasted
- 1 TBL cumin
- 1 TBL chili powder
- 2 tsp paprika
- 1 tsp turmeric
- dash of black pepper
- 1 tsp sea salt
- 1 tsp garlic powder

- 1 onion, chopped and sauteed
- ½ cup almond meal

Instructions:

- sauté onions, translucent
- roast walnuts on stove
- blend walnuts and spices in food processor to mealy consistency
- blend or mash black beans 3/4 of the way, leave 1/4 whole beans
- add the rest of the ingredients to the black beans in a bowl and mix together
- one handful of mixture makes about 8 patties
- grill on bbq or bake in oven at 350 for 40 minutes or cook on stove top in a frying pan for 3 to 4 minutes on each side

Fish, Wild Caught vs Farmed Fish

It's important to know that farm raised fish of ALL species can spell disaster for your health in a number of ways. Just like you need an optimal diet to be healthy, all other animals need their optimal diet as well. And fish were never meant to eat corn, grains, or poultry and pork for that matter. In addition to this unnatural diet, farmed fish of all species are also given a concoction of vitamins, antibiotics, and depending on the fish, synthetic pigments to make up for the lack of natural flesh coloration due to the altered diet. Without it, the flesh of caged salmon, for example, would be an unappetizing, pale gray. The fish are also fed pesticides, along with compounds such as toxic copper sulfate, which is frequently used to keep nets free of algae.

Because of the crowded conditions in which farm raised fish are raised, they are routinely treated with antibiotics to help prevent infection. Not only does this raise concern for residual antibiotic in the fish itself, but the use of antibiotics in this manner helps contribute to the ability of bacteria becoming more and more resistant to the very antibiotics we rely on to combat serious infectious diseases.

The notion that somehow fish farming is more "sustainable" makes absolutely no sense at all. For every pound of salmon for instance, it takes 2-3 pounds of fish chow made from other fish like sardines, mackerel, anchovies, or herring. This needs to be factored into the equation as stocks of the fish used to sustain the fish farms are well on their way to becoming depleted. A logo to look for, when purchasing seafood, is the Marine Stewardship Council logo. Buying products with this logo ensures it was responsibly sourced.

Seek out wild caught fish whenever possible, and be sure to check labels. Don't be fooled by names like "Atlantic Salmon." While you might think that Atlantic salmon means the fish was harvested from the Atlantic Ocean, almost all Atlantic salmon is actually farm-raised.

When you see the Best Aquaculture Practices Certified logo, you know you're getting responsibly farmed fish. BAP certifies the entire production chain: farms, feed mills, hatcheries and processing plants.

Dairy

Many people believe that they must consume dairy in order to build strong bones, but that's not what research is showing. According to a Nurses' Health Study, drinking milk and consuming dairy doesn't reduce fracture risk, in fact, it may increase the risk.

The majority of humans naturally stop producing significant amounts of lactase, the enzyme needed to properly metabolize lactose, sometime between the ages of two and five. Most mammals stop producing the enzymes after they have been weaned. Our bodies just weren't made to digest milk on a regular basis. Most scientists agree that it's better for us to get calcium, potassium, protein, and fats from other food sources, like whole plant foods.

The mass produced, pasteurized, homogenized milk we have in our grocery stores today is not the same milk our ancestors drank.

Conventional Dairy Products

Conventional and organic dairy cattle are raised differently. There are significant differences in the feed and medicines allowed in each. These differences are important because residual pesticides and medicines can be passed from the cow to their milk.

Conventional dairy, found in grocery stores, is filled with antibiotics, hormones, and steroids all of which can cause significant harm to your health. Here are some of the dangers of consuming conventional milk and dairy products:

- Hormone Exposure: Many dairy products are filled with hormones including pituitary, steroid, hypothalamic, and thyroid hormones. When you consume milk that's been pumped with hormones, you risk throwing your own hormonal balance off.
- rBGH (Recombinant Bovine Growth Hormone): You have likely seen rBGH printed on dairy milk products and many products are now striving to be rBGH-free, but not all products. This is a hormone that is injected into cows in order to increase their milk production. The problem with this hormone is that it's genetically engineered and has been linked to various cancers including breast, and colon cancer.
- Antibiotics: This has become a very common concern when it comes to conventional dairy products. Antibiotics,

in general, can be extremely damaging to gut health and when you consume antibiotics via dairy products on a regular, or maybe even daily basis you risk compromising many aspects of your health. Cows are given antibiotics because many of the conventionally fed cows are so sick they have to be pumped with drugs in order to keep producing milk. These drugs then wind up in your daily glass of milk.

Organic Dairy Products

Organic dairy farming in the U.S. really is different from conventional, most of the time (of course there are exceptions). More often than not, dairy in the U.S. comes from crowded, commercial farms where the animals rarely, if ever, go outside. Over 50% of the milk produced comes from just 3% of farms. Most cows (80-90%) don't graze on pasture; instead they eat grain feed made from corn, soy and cottonseed (which is nearly always genetically modified and laden with pesticides).

Organic dairy cattle must be pastured and housed on land that qualifies for organic certification. They must have access to pasture during the entire grazing season and have at least 120 days grazing on pasture to be certified organic.

The USDA guidelines for organic dairy cattle management require preventative health practices to minimize infections and infestations in the herds. However, they also provide and require treatment options in the event that a dairy cow has a life-threatening illness.

If an organic dairy cow has a life threatening infection, or is suffering, antibiotics must be administered. However, the milk from the cow may not be sold or fed to organic calves, and the cow must be transferred to a non-organic dairy farm.

Administration of synthetic hormones to encourage growth or increase milk output is prohibited in organic dairy cattle.

Organic Raw Dairy Products

Raw dairy and full-fat dairy products have proven to contain some powerful health benefits, and don't contain all of the harmful additives like conventional dairy products do.

The first reason why raw milk is a much better option is the fact that these cows are fed what they would naturally eat in the wild. They eat grass, not grains. Since these cows are grazing on grass, they have higher amounts of conjugated linoleic acid (CLA) as well as essential fatty acids in their raw milk products.

Choosing raw milk ensures that you are not consuming milk from a cow that's been fed food so far removed from what their bodies could naturally tolerate. This eliminates the need for antibiotics, steroids, as well as other drugs.

Here are some of the other health benefits of consuming raw milk:

- Tolerance: Many people who have a hard time digesting conventional dairy products do better with raw dairy. While the reason behind this is not entirely clear, The Weston A. Price Foundation found that 80% of 700 families who had been dealing with lactose intolerance no longer had any issues with dairy when they switched to raw milk.
- The Benefits for Children: Many studies in Europe have found that introducing raw milk during childhood could have impressive health benefits in the protection against asthma, and allergies. Again, the exact reason behind this is unknown; speculation is that one reason could be the higher amounts of omega-3 fatty acids found in raw full-fat milk as well as antimicrobial benefits not present in conventional milk options.

- Higher Levels of Fat-Soluble Vitamins: Another surprising benefit of raw milk is its concentration of fat-soluble vitamins, which are important for both heart health as well as cancer prevention. Fat-soluble vitamins also help to balance hormones naturally.
- Excellent Source of Butyrate: Butyrate is a short chain fatty acid which has been shown to help assist in conditions related to inflammation, and metabolism. Not only that, but the CLA levels in raw milk have been shown to help reduce body fat as well as lower high cholesterol levels.

Plant Based Milks

Plant-based milks are quite variable in what they contain. Generally speaking, they grind a bean or nut then add water. The amount of water determines the consistency. Flavors, vitamins, minerals, etc. are added. Commercial plant-based milks are manufactured and can have a variety of additives. I urge consumers to read the label to determine what's best for them.

Making your own plant based milk is the best option. It is easy, quick, fresh and delicious. There are many nuts used which give a variety of flavors to suit your needs; almonds, cashews, hazelnuts, macadamia nuts, pistachios, walnuts, brazil nuts, pecans, pine nuts, etc.

Homemade Nut Milk

makes 1 quart

Ingredients:

- 1-2 cups raw unsalted organic nuts
- 4 cups filtered or purified water

Optional:

- pinch of himalayan sea salt
- 1-2 tablespoon local raw honey or other sweetener
- 1 vanilla bean or 1 teaspoon vanilla extract

Directions:

1. Soak your nuts and vanilla bean (if you are using one) for the appropriate amount of time.
2. Discard soaking water and rinse your nuts and the vanilla bean.
3. Place soaked nuts, the whole soaked vanilla bean (you can chop it up or split it open if you wish) or vanilla extract, honey (or other sweetener), a dash of sea salt and 4 cups of water in a blender. Cover and blend on high for 1-2 minutes. It will be milky and have a bit of foam on the top.
4. Strain milk through a nut bag and squeeze into a bowl.

NOTES:

- These same instructions work for any nut that you prefer to use.
- Store in a covered glass jar, bottle or pitcher in the refrigerator, it'll be good for about 4-5 days.
- Separation is totally natural with homemade nut milks, just be sure to shake it up just before serving.
- I find that 1 cup of nuts is more than enough for 1 quart of milk, some people prefer 2 cups.
- Many variations and flavors of seed and nut milk recipes are easily available online.

Choosing Your Milk

This isn't just about supporting local, organic farmers. It's about knowing what is in our food before that food goes into our bodies. As the saying goes, we are what we eat. You don't want to be stuffed to the gills with artificial chemicals, hormones and additives.

As far as milk and milk alternatives go, your focus should be on overall nutritional benefits. Those benefits vary between the types of milk listed above, and also the brands of milk. For example, one store bought almond milk will have more or less nutritional benefits than the other. As a general rule, avoid added sugars and flavors and choose organic, non-GMO milks.

Getting Enough Calcium

Getting enough calcium is essential to health, and not just bone health. We also need calcium for heart health, nerve signaling as well as muscle contractions.

The great news is that if you choose to keep raw dairy out of your diet, as well as the toxic conventional milk products, there are ways you can get that 600 mg of calcium into your daily diet.

Here are some great sources of calcium that don't include dairy:

- Dark leafy greens
- Blackstrap molasses
- Sesame seeds
- Almonds

Essential Fat

Essential Fatty Acids are an important part of a balanced diet. Increase your intake & you will feel a lot better. Omega-3's are essential fatty acids, which means we have to get them from the food we eat. Omega-3's can help lower both cholesterol and blood pressure, are anti-inflammatory and promote immunity as well as aiding brain function, joint health and mood. There are some excellent plant food sources of Omega-3's and you should include these in your diet; flax seeds, chia seeds, walnuts, tofu, Brussels sprouts, avocados and navy beans. Fish sources include salmon, herring and tuna.

Nature Doesn't Make Bad Fats, Factories Do

Processed seed and vegetable oils became recognized as health foods. Humans only started consuming them about a 100 years ago, because we didn't have the technology to process them until then.

These oils, which include soybean, corn and cottonseed oils, are very high in polyunsaturated Omega-6 fatty acids, which are harmful in excess and can contribute to inflammation. Yet, somehow the nutrition geniuses figured that these would somehow be very healthy for humans and certainly better than the "dangerous" saturated fats which have been eaten from the beginning of time.

Despite decades of anti-fat propaganda, saturated fat has never been proven to cause heart disease. In fact, saturated fat improves some of the most important risk factors for heart disease.

When focusing on unhealthy fats, a good place to start is eliminating your consumption of trans fats. A trans fat is a normal fat molecule that has been twisted and deformed during a process called hydrogenation. During this process, liquid vegetable oil is heated and combined with hydrogen gas. Partially hydrogenating vegetable oils makes them more stable and less likely to spoil, which is very good for food manufacturers and very bad for you. No amount of trans fats is healthy. Even though consumption has gone down, trans fats are still found in processed foods and the FDA still categorizes them as "Generally Regarded as Safe" (GRAS).

Margarine is an unhealthy fake food produced in factories, usually containing trans fats and processed vegetable oils. Butter is a much healthier choice, especially if it comes from grass-fed cows, but should be eaten sparingly.

Fat from whole plants; avocado, coconut, olives, nuts and seeds are the healthiest for the body.

Eggs

Eggs were demonized because of the high amount of cholesterol, but new studies show that they don't raise cholesterol in the blood or contribute to heart disease. Eggs are among the most nutritious foods on the planet. Telling people to ditch the yolks may be just be the most ridiculous nutrition advice in history.

One of the lesser-known benefits of eggs is its impact on cognitive health, primarily due to the high levels of choline present. Choline is often grouped with B-vitamins, but in fact, it is a somewhat unknown nutrient that helps to create critical neural pathways in the brain. About 90% of the population is estimated to get less choline than the body requires, but whole eggs supply choline in large quantities.

The diet that the hen has will obviously be reflected in the nutrient content of the egg. For that reason, it is a far better choice to consume free range, pasture-fed eggs, as they have consistently been shown to have higher omega-3 content, vitamin E content, tend to be larger, and are more densely packed with nutrients.

Choosing Your Water

When choosing water for yourself and your family, you want to ensure that the water you choose is safe (free of bacteria and chemicals), clear and colorless and has no unpleasant odor. Yet with a myriad of options available, including bottled waters, charcoal filters and in-home systems, choosing the healthiest water can be a confusing task.

There are several types of water to choose from. The worst water to drink is tap water. Tap water, also known as utility water, runs through extensive piping prior to coming out of your faucet. It is often treated with chlorine to kill off unwanted bacteria and may also contain lead or aluminum and added fluoride. In terms of water quality, I do not recommend drinking unfiltered tap water due to the presence of numerous impurities. Legally, municipal water has to be safe to drink and bathe in, so drinking it will not harm you. But this does not mean that your drinking water is entirely free of contaminants or additives that can contribute to adverse tastes and odors.

Distilled water is now causing some controversy as some claim that it leaches minerals from the body and is overly acidic. The body does not thrive in a state of acidity; bacteria, fungi and viruses proliferate in an acidic environment.

Similar to distilled water, reverse osmosis water produces demineralized water with an acidic pH. Some recent reports claim that prolonged consumption of distilled or demineralized water can lead to various forms of mineral deficiency.

Bottled water isn't just bad for the health of our planet, it has a detrimental effect on our own bodies. Water bottles contain chemicals like BPA that can cause reproductive issues, asthma and dizziness. Studies even suggest a possible risk of breast cancer. Bottled water is tested for microbes and other water pollution four times less than tap water. Some of the large water brands have admitted that their bottled water is nothing more than filtered tap water. Water packaged in disposable bottles is shockingly expensive when compared to other sources of drinkable water. For the recommended amount of eight glasses of water a day, bottled water costs:

- $1,800 a year
- 26 times more than a filtered pitcher
- 3,675 times more than tap water

Most experts say that most tap water is actually safer than bottled.

Water ionizers can be purchased and connected directly to a faucet at your sink. Water first passes through a multistage granular activated carbon filter that removes chlorine, metals, sediments and various volatile compounds. The filter also contains silver to prevent bacterial growth. Ionized water is alkaline, not acidic.

Spring water is widely accepted to be the cleanest water on earth; provided its has been sourced naturally and not subjected to transportation factors such as pumps, pipes, faucets or BPA-laden bottles.

Some store-bought spring water is bottled and some aren't filtered at all. Try to find local spring water source because it often contains beneficial elements like magnesium, potassium, and calcium, water is meant to come out of the ground clean, and that's how we're supposed to drink it.

The best type of water to drink is naturally filtered, mineral rich water from wells, natural springs and natural underground mineral water reservoirs. These types of water are living water and contain minerals such as potassium, sodium and magnesium, all vital for helping your body perform optimally.

The safest water to drink in most areas is filtered water. Water filters not only help improve the flavor of your water but also protect you from impurities such as rust particles and harmful contaminants such as bacteria and lead. There are pitchers, counter top, faucet, under the sink and whole house water filters. There are many systems to choose from, buy the best one you can afford. Any water filter is better than none.

We cannot survive more than a few days on earth without water. Its ready supply is too easily taken for granted. As pressure increases on our supply, pressure from people, industrial processes and pollutants, water is in grave danger of becoming just another commodity in the market place, and supplies are dominated by the rich and powerful. In the traditional world, in religion and even in municipal engineering, water has always been seen as a common resource, indivisible as air. Equity demands that it remains so. Be mindful where your water comes from, the quality of it and who you are giving your money to.

Become a Divine Feminine Conscious Eater

Transitioning off the Standard American Diet can be hard for most people. Take your time, and be gentle with yourself. Weather your goal is to be plant predominant, vegetarian, vegan or raw, it is about peace, and the first place to start is to be peaceful with yourself during the transition.

Most people can deal with change if it is gradual. If the change comes too quickly, it then becomes a shock to the system. Usually, the complete transition takes several years. In the overall picture, how long the process takes doesn't matter. What matters is that you have chosen to move along the divine path toward health, harmony, and peace. Keep this in mind as you create your own Divine Feminine Diet eating plan that suits your lifestyle and level of commitment.

Set yourself a long term goal and short term goals to get you there. If your goals were to eventually be an organic raw food vegan, your plan might look like this:

- Step One is setting a time line to transition from your current diet to natural, organic, whole foods. This means letting go of all processed, irradiated, chemicalized, pesticide-ridden and fungicide-containing, adulterated, fast, and junk foods. In this stage you may begin to give up red meats.

- Step Two is letting go of all flesh foods, such as poultry and fish. It also includes not eating eggs.
- Step Three is a vegetarian diet with the inclusion of dairy at the beginning and then moving to an 80% live-food intake by the end.
- Step Four is vegan without dairy and may be as much as 95% to 100% live foods by the end.

Whichever divine life style you are aiming for, set your goals accordingly and go slow and steady, being accountable but also kind and patient with yourself and never forget your sense of humor.

Visualization

- See yourself as strong and healthy, free of pain or sickness, with a pure spirit and Goddess-like mind.
- Now close your eyes and breathe in radiant health and exhale all negativity and sickness. Do this several times.
- Now see the new "you" as a conscious eater. Take as long as you need to pray or meditate until such a vision of your divine potential appears.
- Feel the experience of this vision in your body as you are filled with health, spiritual power, and sensitivity.
- Express the emotions and thoughts associated with the new "you" as a conscious eater.

Use Your Common Sense

When my clients are unsure what they should eat when they desire to live a healthier lifestyle I tell them to use their intuition and common sense and ask themselves "Did people eat this 100 or 200 years ago?" and "If I had to live off of the land, out in nature, as nature intended it to be.....:

- What would be available to eat?
- How would I prepare it?
- How much of it would I eat?
- What would be my medicine?"

Your answers will differ depending on what part of the world and climate you live in. Remember, science is in it infancy, Mother Nature is Supreme. You are a child of nature, you are made of nature.

This is what I know:

- Our bodies are the same bodies that our ancient ancestors had, evolution has not changed our bodies or the nutritional requirements the body needs for vibrant health.
- We have ancient bodies living in an artificial modern world, which is making us ill.
- We can't completely return back to the wild, so we have to find a healthy balance between ancient wisdom and our modern world to survive and thrive.

The answer to all health challenges is always:

- Eat more real food
- Drink more water
- Use nature's medicines

- Get outside and back in touch with nature
- Love yourself enough to make changes
- Believe in your divinity and the power of your soul which has the power to heal your body

Real foods are anything we ate prior to "civilization" before we learned to "improve food" by processing it, mass produce it and package it to last forever. Real food includes organic everything; fruit, nuts and seeds, vegetables, greens, herbs, whole grains, grass-fed, free range meats and eggs and wild caught fish. The vitamins, minerals, fats, amino acids and all the nutrients we need for healing will be in these foods.

This is not to say you have to eat only these foods to the exclusion of all others; you just have to add more of them to your current diet. Once you are nourishing your body it will no longer want to be fat. As a result, your body will start to prefer real foods to dead, processed, refined, artificial varieties we've become accustomed to eating.

Your body interprets lack of essential nutrients as a form of famine. Once your body starts to understand that fake foods are starving and poisoning you, your body will start to reject them and crave real food. I didn't believe this until it happened to me and I started craving salad after not having one for a few days. I would have never in my life "craved" a salad!

Once you consider our ancient ancestors diet, look inward and use your intuition and common sense and listen to your body, you will not just survive, but thrive as you adjust your diet accordingly.

When you decide to eat organic plant based food you take your Goddess power back by deciding for yourself what you are going to put in your body. Rather than feeling deprived by saying no to junk food, you will feel empowered that you give a damn about yourself. Permanent health and weight loss is eating better not less. Eating a plant-based diet will certainly be an upgrade for your health, both physical and mental.

CHAPTER 4

Bring Love Back Into the Kitchen

"At feasts, remember that you are entertaining two guests: body and soul. What you give to the body, you presently lose, what you give to the soul, you keep forever." Epictetus

Processed foods are not made with love. How could they be? Factories churn out hundreds, if not thousands of nearly identical processed items each day and all or most of the seasoning, cooking and stirring is done by machines.

Processed food companies do not have the optimal wellness of their consumers in mind, its all about profits. Therefore, many companies use inexpensive ingredients and pump their products full of chemical additives to enhance flavor, color, texture and prolong the shelf life. The result of so many people turning to processed foods as their main diet are without doubt linked to chronic illnesses and obesity.

Homemade foods made in your own kitchen have completely the opposite effect. Making meals at home just seems to make everyone happy. Do you remember the last time you made a loved one their favorite meal and their eyes just lit up? And do you remember the last time you all ate together as a family and how special it was? Sitting down and eating a meal that you created together is a daily celebration of love.

- Home cooking allows you to come together, with your family and friends at home or college or wherever you live or are visiting.
- It's about finding a way to connect with your community.
- Good food is the greatest gift of gratitude you can give your body.

We live in a culture where parents were never taught how to cook as a child and don't cook as adults. They aren't teaching their children to cook and turn to fast food or commercially prepared food for themselves and their families. Cooking homemade food isn't just about physical health, it's about connecting with each other. Learn how to cook and spend time in the kitchen and at the table with the people in your life, even if it is only for a few days a week to begin with. If you live alone, love your Divine Feminine self enough to cook for yourself and show your divine body some love.

Ancient women put a special sacred meaning in everything they were doing. Cooking, embroidery towels, brushing their hair, etc. was a magical ritual. Everything that women did, they charged with their energy through their prayers and manifestations.

It is time to bring love back into the kitchen. You don't have to spend hours slaving over a hot stove. There are plenty of nutritious, yummy meals that can be made in just minutes. It is the quality, intent and the care that are key.

Honor Your Kitchen Space

- Begin by cleaning your kitchen and removing clutter that doesn't belong.
- Light a candle or incense.
- Bring in a vase of flowers or fresh herbs.
- Say a prayer or blessing to dedicate your cooking area as a sacred space.
- Make your kitchen the heart of the home again.
- Remember to be patient with yourself as you are learning to cook with love, trying new recipes and being mindful of preparing nutritious meals.
- Limit your distractions while you are cooking and creating in the kitchen. Talking on the phone, watching TV and thinking of the days problems will distract you from the practice of cooking with love.

Gratitude

Ancient native people believed that everything had a spirit, and they understood the importance of communicating with the life force in all things. For example, they would ask for blessings from the Spirit of the Sea before fishing, or they would ask for support from the Spirit of Rain for their crops. Plants were honored before they were harvested. Before the hunt, hunters would give thanks to the Spirit of the animal being hunted and ask forgiveness for the life that was taken.

To our peril we take food for granted and don't give much thought to what it is, where it came from or how it was grown, raised or killed. One of the most powerful mind shifts we can have is to realize preparing fresh food for ourselves and our families is a privilege to celebrate not an inconvenience to dread.

Spirituality Of Food

By re-adopting our ancestors plant-based diet, you'll be assisting in the reconfiguration of your spiritual tie to Mother Earth. When you strengthen that spiritual tie, your mind will operate with more clarity, empowering you to think with a Divine Feminine mindset.

Natural, whole food is organic matter that is made up of energy, just like everything else, because it is created by the earth's soil, it exists at a higher vibration than something that is created by a factory. As a result of being whole and organic, natural foods are more reactive to good thoughts you send towards it, as thoughts are also a form of energy. When there is emotion behind your thought, a physical manifestation will soon follow. Our ancestors understood this and that is why they always prayed over their food and water. We should continue this practice.

Conversely, processed foods resonate at a low vibration.

Prepare Your Food With Love

Energetically, love is the rock star of our highest vibration, it's what we ideally should be operating from. And because we radiate love at higher vibrations, we attract love in return. Our aura is healthy, and we acknowledge that we are joy and are experiencing joy. Your energy, love and joy will be infused into the food you are preparing.

Organization Eliminates Frustration

It is hard to feel peace and love when you are frustrated in the kitchen. Make a plan and follow your plan.

- Organize your pantry, cupboards, drawers, fridge, and freezer

- Stock your kitchen with nutritious food
- Once a week make a weekly menu plan for the following week
- Make a shopping list and get every ingredient you need on your menu
- Every evening make a menu for the following day and write it down.
- Wash your dishes and clean your kitchen every single day.

Raise the Vibrational Energy of Your Food

Prepare your meals with love and eat with gratitude. Say a prayer or grace before eating. Blessing your food may be considered old school thinking, but I think it works like this: it binds us together in reverence and gratitude for our mother, the earth, it revives the 'old ways' of creating blessings for ourselves, our family, community and the planet herself, and it reconnects us with the joy of nourishing and being nourished.

Eat mindfully and enjoy the colors, shapes, tastes, textures, and aromas of your food. Believe that you are receiving nourishment and healing from your meal. This practice will raise the vibrational energy of your food even when it isn't the most perfect food all of the time.

Women's Relationship With Food

Once, women were honored as strong, beautiful, creative, sensual beings. The feminine aspect of life was necessary for our very survival, and the sacred feminine was honored by ancients around the world as the bringer of life. Woman was life itself. The power of women in those ancient times was undeniable, without women, we humans would not be here now.

As male dominance succeeded in stripping women of their

power and spiritual heritage, civilizations also lost their connection to Mother Earth. Skills women possessed, once considered sacred, have been turned over to industry, mass production, and big business. It was the shift to ownership of crop and land (usually by an elite class of landholders and the Church) that spelled the end of the goddess and her gift economy. In order for the new capitalistic order to succeed, women's role in food production and their spiritual authority had to be removed. Women's traditional access to land, and control over the crops they cultivated was replaced by a labor force.

From our earliest days as hunter-gatherers to the first domestication of plants, it was women who stoked the first hearths, stirred the first pots, brewed the first beer, and baked the first bread.

Women's role in food production was considered sacred. Women were linked with food not only because they cultivated and prepared it, but also because their own bodies, like the Great Goddess, were a source of food and life.

The vast bulk of historical evidence suggests that women were the primary gatherers, introducing the deliberate cultivation of plants and the various complex processes such as cooking, baking, preservation and food storage, basketry, and pottery that went along with it.

Long before food was bought and sold for profit, no act of food production, from harvesting, growing, preparing, preserving, storing, cooking or baking was left unblessed by women's prayers, rituals and devotions. And for most of human history nearly every domestic activity from making pots to planting seeds to baking bread was ritual "hearthcraft". To put it very simply, women's food magic had one central purpose, to honor and nourish the great mother of all, who in turn nourished them.

Food is no longer freely given by the earth but bought at the store. What was once gathered, grown, harvested, prepared and consumed with ritual, ceremony and devotion, is now a product devoid of spiritual meaning.

Women no longer gather communally to harvest with prayer and song, but shop harried and alone in corporate superstores, and the kitchen is a place where we consume the processed and fast foods that suit our busy lifestyles.

Women today are suffering from an internal conflict, in which our hidden hungers, the sensual pleasures of food and cooking are all too often obscured by the increasing demands of careers, families, battles over body image, and the desire for a life outside the "traditional" domain of the kitchen.

It's no wonder why we are perpetually dieting, suffering from eating disorders, and have an obsession with "watching what we eat". Modern women have such a complicated relationship with food. We must be careful not to develop an unhealthy obsession with healthy eating, trading one compulsion for another.

Despite our association with food and cooking, the kitchen is often viewed as disempowering drudgery, this wasn't always the case. Growing evidence in the fields of anthropology suggests that long before women ate last at the table and maintained their trim figures, long before cooking was part of an invisible unpaid economy, women had control over the crops they harvested, cultivated, cooked and consumed.

Cooking is the essential human activity at the heart of all cultures. By relying upon corporations to process our food we've disrupted our essential link to the natural world. We need to reclaim our lost food traditions and revel again in the magical activity of making food.

The kitchen is a holy place where the gifts of nature are transformed into physical, emotional, and even spiritual forms of sustenance. We need to forge a deeper, more meaningful connection to the ingredients and cooking techniques that we use to nourish ourselves.

Food is Magical and Sacred

- Develop a healthy relationship with healthy food and your goddess body.
- Buy the best ingredients you can. Prepare and season them to your hearts content.
- Your food should taste good, look good, smell good and make you happy.
- One of the most enjoyable things in life is real, delicious food, especially when enjoyed with others.
- Whenever you eat, do so with gratitude in your heart and with the intention that your food is going to heal and nourish you. Tell your body to absorb what it needs and discard the rest. Your body hears you and believes what you tell it.

Connecting to our ancient selves is a medicine that can heal us in this modern day.

CHAPTER 5

Plant Medicine/Remedies

Your body is not a problem to fix,
it is a miracle to discover.

Human beings and plants have co-evolved for millions of years, so it makes perfect sense that our complex bodies would be adapted to absorb needed, beneficial compounds from complex plants and ignore the rest. This is an established fact in nutrition. Plant medicines are plants whose properties provide medicinal value to us. We seem to think that drinking herbs that the earth offers to cure a sore throat, for gas and bloating, for heart health, or physical related illnesses is ok. What we're forgetting is that we are more than just physical beings. We are also emotional, spiritual and intellectual beings. Humans ingest far beyond just a physical level. So it makes sense that the earth would also provide us with medicinal plants to help heal our emotional, spiritual and intellectual aspects.

The natural world is full of beauty, sustenance, and healing if you only know where to look. For hundreds of thousands of years, human cultures around the globe had all of their needs met by plants, animals, and natural resources that surrounded them. For medicine, they could find a finely stocked pharmacy in the roots, herbs, fungi, and trees all around them. Some of these early peoples discovered that some plant medicines did not just heal toothaches and other physical ailments but expanded the mind in incredible ways as well. They placed these sacred plants at the heart of their spiritual traditions.

Unfortunately, in current day society, we have moved far away from this perspective. Plants are rarely viewed as anything more than objects that can be reduced to a chemical component, or an object that looks nice perched in a corner. However, as with many aspects of our natural world, there is so much more to plants than meets the eye.

Herbs

Medicinal Herbs have been in use from the beginning of time and are renowned for their effectiveness in many diseases. These natural herbs are very effective in boosting the immune system, increasing the body resistance to infections, healing the allergies, and raising and renewing the body vitality. Many people have started to resort to herbal remedies for diseases and as a result, they have started growing herbs in their garden. Besides making tinctures, creams and salves you can add fresh herbs to your meals, smoothies, juices, broths and salads.

The remarkable aspect of herbs is their combination of several different healing properties. Thus, each herb will have a combination of specific effects on particular systems of the body, and also some very general effects. By carefully matching the herbal properties with the symptoms being treated, it is possible to confront the entire scope of the disease at once, achieving a remedy quickly and with the minimum possible dosage. Also, by referencing the herbal properties, it becomes easier to substitute one herb for another.

Alteratives:

Also known as blood purifiers, these agents gradually and favorably alter the condition of the body. They are used in treating toxicity of the blood, infections, arthritis, cancer and skin eruptions.

Some Alteratives include: Red Clover, Echinacea, Dandelion Root, Alfalfa, Marshmallow Root, Black Walnut Bark, Burdock, Calendula Flower, Ginseng, Licorice, Raspberry Leaf, Wheatgrass Powder,White Willow Bark, and Nettle Leaf.

Analgesics:

Herbs that are taken to relieve pain. Some Analgesics include: Echinacea, Chamomile, Ginger, Lemongrass, Noni Fruit, Skullcap, Turmeric, White Willow Bark, and Valerian.

Antacids:

Herbs that neutralize excess acids in the stomach and intestines. Many also have demulcent properties to protect the stomach lining. Some Antacids are Dandelion Root, Slippery Elm Bark, and Kelp.

Antiabortives:

Herbs that help to inhibit abortive tendencies. The herbs will not interfere with the natural process of miscarriage when the fetus is damaged or improperly secured. Antiabortives include: Kelp.

Antiasthmatics:

Herbs that relieve the symptoms of asthma. Some, like Lobelia, are strong Antispasmodics that dilate the bronchioles. Others, like Yerba Santa help break up the mucus. Some herbs like Mullein may be smoked for quick relief, which may also be taken as tea. Other Antiasthmatics include Açai Berry Juice, Ginseng, Rooibos African Red Tea, and Wild Cherry Bark.

Antibiotics:

Substances that inhibit the growth of, or destroy, bacteria, viruses or amoebas. While many herbal antibiotics have direct germ killing effects, they have as a primary action, the stimulation of the body's own immune response. Excessive use of antibiotics will eventually destroy the beneficial bacteria of the intestines. In fighting stubborn infections it is a good idea to maintain favorable intestinal flora by eating miso, tamari, or fresh yogurt. Important antibiotic herbs include Echinacea and Olive Leaf.

Anticatarrhals:

Herbs that eliminate or counteract the formation of mucus. A treatment for catarrh should also include the use of herbs that aid elimination through sweat (diaphoretics), urine (diuretics), and feces (laxatives). Anticatarrhal herbs include: Cayenne Pepper, Ginkgo Biloba, Sage, Cinnamon, Mullein, Wild Cherry Bark, and Yerba Santa.

Antipyretics:

Cooling herbs used to reduce or prevent fevers. Cooling may refer to neutralizing harmful acids in the blood (excess heat) as well as reducing body temperature. Antipyretics include: Alfalfa, Skullcap, Dulse, Rosemary, White Willow Bark, and Kelp.

Antiseptics:

Herbs that can be applied to the skin to prevent the growth of bacteria. This includes the Astringents. Some Antiseptics include: Calendula, Astragalus, Chamomile, Hibiscus Flower, Nettle Leaf, Olive Leaf, Rosehips, Rosemary, Turmeric, White Willow Bark, Yerba Santa, and Sage.

Antispasmodics:

Herbs that prevent or relax muscle spasms. They may be applied either internally or externally for relief. Antispasmodics are included in most herb formulas to relax the body and allow it to use its full energy for healing. Some Antispasmodics include: Astragalus, Cayenne Pepper, Chamomile, Eleutherococcus, Skullcap, Hibiscus Flower, Hops, Lavender, Lemon Balm, Licorice, Mullein Leaf, Nettle Leaf, Valerian, Passionflower, Peppermint, Red Clover, Rosehips, Sage, Spearmint Leaf, Yerba Santa, and Raspberry Leaf.

Aphrodisiacs:

Substances used to improve sexual potency and power. Aphrodisiacs include: Astragalus, Burdock, Ginseng, and Maca Root.

Astringents:

Herbs that have a constricting or binding effect. They are commonly used to check hemorrhages and secretions, and to treat swollen tonsils and hemorrhoids. The main herbal Astringents contain tannins, which are found in most plants, especially in tree barks. Important Astringents include: Aloe Vera, Apple Fiber, Beet Root, Calendula, Cayenne Pepper, Cinnamon, Dandelion Root, Eyebright, Fenugreek, Hawthorn Berry, Hibiscus Flower, Mullein Leaf, Olive Leaf, Peppermint, Raspberry Leaf, Rosehips, Rosemary, Sage, St. John's Wort, White Willow Bark, Wild Cherry Bark, and Yucca Root.

Carminatives:

Herbs and spices taken to relieve gas and griping (severe pains in the bowels). Examples of Carminatives include: Astragalus, Cayenne Pepper, Chamomile, Cinnamon, Cloves, Ginger, Ginseng, Lavender, Lemon Balm, Lemongrass, Peppermint, Sage, Valerian, Wild Cherry Bark, and Yerba Santa.

Cholagogues:

Substances used to promote the flow and discharge of bile into the small intestine. These will also be laxatives, as the bile will stimulate elimination. Some Cholagogues are: Aloe Vera, Dandelion Root, Licorice, Red Clover, Wormwood, and Yerba mate.

Demulcents:

Soothing substances, usually mucilage, taken internally to protect damaged or inflamed tissues. Usually a Demulcent herb will be used along with diuretics to protect the kidney and urinary tract, especially when kidney stones and gravel are present. Important Demulcents include: Apple Fiber, Burdock, Cinnamon, Dulse, Fenugreek, Ginseng, Kelp, Marshmallow Root, Milk Thistle, Mullein Leaf, Slippery Elm Bark, Licorice, and Oat Straw.

Diaphoretics:

Herbs used to induce sweating. To administer Diaphoretics effectively, the stomach and bowels should be emptied by fasting and using an enema. However, laxatives should not be used before using these herbs. Sweating teas should be hot; when given cold, they act as diuretics. Some Diaphoretics include: Burdock, Calendula, Cayenne Pepper, Chamomile, Elder Berries, Ginger, Lemon Balm, Peppermint, Rosemary, and Spearmint Leaf.

Diuretics:

Herbs that increase the flow of urine. They are used to treat water retention, obesity, lymphatic swellings, nerve inflammations such as lumbago and sciatica, infections of the urinary tract, skin eruptions, and kidney stones. Whenever a Diuretic is given, a lesser amount of Demulcent herb is also given to buffer the effect of the diuretic on the kidneys (especially when the Diuretic contains irritating properties) and to protect the tissues from the movement of kidney stones. Some Diuretics include: Alfalfa, Astragalus, Beet Root, Elder Berries, Hibiscus Flower, Marshmallow, Nettle Leaf, Burdock, Dandelion, Hops, Oat Straw, Red Clover, Yerba mate, and Hawthorn Berry.

Emmenagogues:

Herbs that promote menstruation, usually causing it to occur earlier, and sometimes with increased flow. These have been used in the past to induce abortions, so extreme caution is advised. All of these, when taken in sufficient quantity to cause abortion, have other strong effects on the body. None of these should be taken when a woman wants to be pregnant. These are now commonly used to help regulate the menstrual cycle. Herbs with strong Emmenagogue properties include: Pennyroyal, Juniper Berries, and Black Cohosh. Herbs with some emmenagogue properties include: Aloe Vera, Calendula, Chamomile, Lemon Balm, and Nettle Leaf.

Emollients:

Substances that are softening, soothing, and protective to the skin. These include Aloe Vera, Fenugreek, Kelp, Marshmallow Root, and Slippery Elm Bark.

Expectorants:

Herbs that assist in expelling mucus from the lungs and throat. Expectorants include: Eyebright, Fenugreek, Ginseng, Lemongrass, Licorice, Mullein, Nettle Leaf, Red Clover, Slippery Elm Bark, Wild Cherry Bark, Yucca Root and Yerba Santa.

Galactogogues:

Substances that increase the secretion of milk. Anise Seed, Cumin, Dandelion Root, and Fennel.

Hemostatics:

Substances that arrest hemorrhaging. These include astringents and herbs that affect the coagulation of blood. Cayenne Pepper, Mullein, Nettle Leaf, and Raspberry Leaf.

Laxatives:

Herbs that promote bowel movements. A strong laxative that causes increased intestinal peristalsis is called a purgative in many texts. Some laxatives include: Aloe Vera, Black Walnut Bark, Elder Berries, Licorice, Yerba mate, and Yucca Root.

Lithotriptics:

Herbs that help to dissolve and eliminate urinary and biliary stones and gravel. For kidney and bladder stones, use Parsley, Dandelion Root and Nettle Leaf. For the gallbladder, use Wild Cherry Bark and Cascara Sagrada.

Nervines:

Herbs that calm nervous tension and nourish the nervous system. Herbs with nervine properties include: Chamomile, Hops, Passionflower, Rooibos African Red Tea, Rosemary, Skullcap, and Valerian.

Parasiticides:

Herbs that destroy parasites in the digestive tract or on the skin. Parasiticides include: Chamomile, Cinnamon, Cloves, Black Walnut Bark, Nettle Leaf, and Wormwood.

Rubefacients:

Substances that increase the flow of blood at the surface of the skin and produce redness where they are applied. Their function is to draw inflammation and congestion from deeper areas. They are useful for the treatment of arthritis, rheumatism, and other joint problems and for sprains. Rubefacients include: Cayenne Pepper, Cinnamon, Olive Leaf, and Wheatgrass Powder.

Sedatives:

Herbs that strongly quiet the nervous system. These will include antispasmodics and nervines. Useful Sedatives include: Valerian, Hops, Chamomile, Passionflower, St. John's Wort, Wild Cherry Bark and Skullcap.

Sialagogues:

Substances that stimulate the flow of saliva and thus aid in the digestion of starches. Some Sialagogues are Beet Root, Echinacea, Ginger, Licorice, Rooibos African Red Tea, and Yerba Santa.

Stimulants:

Herbs that increase the energy of the body, drive the circulation, break up obstruction and warm the body. Stimulants include: Bee Pollen, Cloves, Cayenne Pepper, Cinnamon, Echinacea, Eleutherococcus, Ginseng, Ginger, Ginkgo Biloba, Rosemary, Sage, Peppermint, Raspberry Leaf, Valerian, Yerba Santa,and Astragalus.

Tonics:

Herbs that promote the functions of the systems of the body. Most Tonics have general effects on the whole body, but also have a marked effect on a specific system. Some tonic herbs include: Açai Berry Juice, Alfalfa, Apple Fiber, Burdock, Cayenne Pepper, Dandelion Root, Fenugreek, Ginseng, Hawthorn Berry, Hops, Milk Thistle, and Yerba mate.

Vulneraries:

Herbs that encourage the healing of wounds by promoting cell growth and repair. Some Vulneraries are: Aloe Vera, Cayenne Pepper, Calendula, Fenugreek, Ginseng, Mullein Leaf, Rosemary, Marshmallow Root, and Slippery Elm Bark.

Flower Essences

Flower remedies are a form of alternative medicine based on the principles of homeopathy. Homeopathy is the belief that the body can cure itself.

Flower essences are the vibrational message of a flower transmitted to water by solarization, and the vibrational resonance of the flower is memorized by the water, used in support of achieving an emotional balance.

Flower essences are liquid extracts used to address profound issues of emotional well-being, soul development, and mind-body health. They are part of an emerging field of subtle energy medicine, which also includes homeopathy, acupuncture, color therapy, therapeutic touch and similar modalities.

Flower essences deliver the subtle energy of plants to our body. It's a form of energy medicine that helps balance our emotional well-being. Flower essences are a powerful tool for shifting mindset, moving through trapped emotions, releasing stored trauma, and improving habitual emotional states .

Essential Oils

Essential oils are the essence of a plant, a gift from the earth, distilled and prepared for you to bring the power of nature into your home.

Inside many plants, hidden in roots, seeds, flowers, bark, are concentrated, highly potent chemical compounds. These natural compounds are essential oils.

Essential oils give a plant its scent, protect it from hazardous environmental conditions, and even assist it with pollination, among other important functions and benefits.

Plant extracts and plant-based products are deeply rooted in the traditions of the past. Essential oils have been used by ancient civilizations across the globe for:

- Aromatherapy
- Personal care
- Healthcare practices
- Religious ceremonies
- Beauty treatments
- Food preparation

CHAPTER 6

What Is Your Body Telling You?

> ***"A person with their health has a thousand dreams. A person without their health has only one, which of course is to get it back."***

The ancients were much more in tune with their bodies and the earth than we are today. Chinese medicine and Ayurvedic medicine, which has been around for over 5,000 years and called the mother of all medicine, still use the signs of the body and bodily functions to diagnose and prevent impeding ailments.

Western medicine puts no stock in these modalities, they call them pseudo- science, pre-science and quackery. However our medical tests can only detect a full blown disease in its end stages. As I mentioned earlier the science of man is constantly changing and evolving so you can't put 100% of your faith in that either.

While the following can't necessarily diagnose diseases, it's extremely useful for understanding which areas of the body the health practitioner should pay attention to and which parts may be at risk for the development of certain ailments.

"It's more important to understand the imbalances in your body's basic systems, and restore balance, rather than name the disease and match a pill to the ill." Mark Hyman M.D.

Reading the Signs of Your Body

Your Finger Nails

Moons: The more energetic a person is, the whiter (and more present) their moons will be. The fewer moons a person has on their nails, the more like likely they are to feel tired and suffer from poor immunity.

It's normal for the pinky nail to have a small or absent moon, but if you find that moons are absent across most of all of your fingers, it's a sign that you may need to support this inner fire that governs your digestion, energy and metabolism.

White Spots: White spots on the nails are very common, mainly due to the fact that more and more people are becoming deficient in minerals such as magnesium, selenium, and zinc.

Zinc deficiency leads to chronically low stomach acid. Low stomach acid means you can't break down and extract the amino acids within the protein you eat. As your zinc levels are replenished, your HCL will increase and you can begin properly digesting protein once again.

Vertical Lines and Ridges: Vertical lines on the nails are extremely common, and often seen as a normal sign of aging. As you age, the efficiency of your blood circulation (especially peripheral circulation to the hands and feet) decreases. This means far less nutrients and oxygen are delivered to the nail, causing the loss of a smooth, hydrated surface (perhaps combined with increased brittleness). If this is happening before your time, the answer may be quite simple:

- increase the amount of nutrients you're taking in
- support digestion so those nutrients can actually be absorbed
- improve circulation so those nutrients can get to the nail where they belong

Young or old, you want your circulation and digestion to be strong so that your blood can bring nutrients to every nook and cranny of your body.

Pail Nails: pale nails are said to be caused by "blood deficiency," which isn't always identical to anemia but certainly can be. If for any reason you become what they consider "deficient in blood," either due to blood loss or poor red blood cell production (low iron and b12), the liver meridian is not able to properly regulate blood flow. This pattern of disharmony not only presents itself as pale nails, but also can include symptoms such as hair loss, dry skin, dry eyes, and brittle nails.

In women, the most telltale sign would be scanty periods that feel incomplete and end too quickly.

The good news is that "blood deficiency" is simply a pattern that practitioners look for and not a disease. Just like its most common cause (iron deficiency), it can be easily corrected with proper habits, nutrition and supplementation if necessary.

Yellow Finger Nails: Nail polish (specifically darker, richer shades) is the most common culprit when fingernails turn yellow, especially when it's affecting the entire nail from top to bottom. Always make sure you're using a clear base polish first to add a layer of protection between your fingernails and the colored polish. Consider taking a break from polish in general until the discoloration subsides.

If this is not the cause and you find your nails are continually getting worse even when abstaining from polish, there are two possibilities you'll want to explore. The first is nail fungus, which is often accompanied by a progressive distortion/deterioration in nail shape and even a foul odor as the infection progresses.

The second is nail psoriasis, which involves the nails detaching or lifting from the nail bed rather than a distortion of shape. You'll notice a chalky white buildup right where the nail is lifting due to hyperkeratosis (an overproduction of keratin, most likely prompted by the underlying inflammation present in autoimmune disorders). There will also be pain present when the nail is lifting due to psoriasis, which doesn't usually happen in the case of nail fungus.

Horizontal Ridges or Groves: These horizontal lines or ridges are called "Beau's lines," named after the French physician Joseph Honoré Simon Beau who first described and researched these grooves in 1846. The most common causes of Beau's lines vary greatly and can include:

- direct injury to the nail matrix
- inflammatory/autoimmune conditions that can affect the nails such as psoriasis
- infection in or around the nail plate
- nutritional deficiencies
- illnesses that are accompanies by high fever (this is sort of the 'mark' it can leave behind)
- metabolic conditions
- certain drugs (especially chemotherapy)
- diminished blood flow to the fingers (often seen in those with Raynaud's)

Unfortunately, Beau's lines are among the least specific nail signs one can encounter, and may be caused by any disease severe enough to disrupt normal nail synthesis. When the body is battling a difficult ailment, it presses "pause" on bodily functions that are not necessary for healing or survival, including nail growth.

However, there are still some clues you can look at to pinpoint the cause, for example: the width of the line is usually a good indicator of the given ailment's duration. Likewise, measuring the distance from the line to where the nail bed begins can give you an approximate time frame of when the ailment or insult may have occurred. Fingernails take about 6 months to regrow completely, so if you see a Beau's line halfway up the nail it means that the problem occurred about 3 months ago.

Blue Nails: A blue face is a clear indication that someone's lacking airflow, and blue nails mean the same thing, you're not getting enough oxygen to your fingertips. This could be caused by respiratory disease or a vascular problem called Raynaud's Disease, which is a rare disorder of the blood vessels. Some people just have slower blood circulation, especially when exposed to cold temperatures, but have a physician check your blood and oxygenation levels if your nails are persistently blue.

White Lines: Horizontal white lines that span the entire nail, are paired, and appear on more than one nail are called Muehrcke's lines. These could be an indication of kidney disease, liver abnormalities, or a lack of protein and other nutrients. They are thought to be caused by a disruption in blood supply to the nail bed because of underlying disease.

Shorter horizontal white marks or streaks, however, are likely just the result of trauma to the base of your nail. These may last from weeks to months and usually will disappear on their own.

Pits and Grooving: Depressions and small cracks in your nails are known as "pitting" of the nail bed and are often associated with psoriasis, an inflammatory disease that leads to scaly or red patches all over the body. Individuals who suffer from psoriasis develop clusters of cells along the nail bed that accumulate and disrupt the linear, smooth growth of a normal nail. As these cells are sloughed off, grooves or depressed areas are left behind on the surface. A physical exam is often all you need for a diagnosis, after which your doctor may recommend topical medications or light therapy.

Your Tongue

We all grew up with every doctors visit beginning with a tongue depressor saying ahhh!

The tongue is the beginning of the digestive tract, which lumbers on another 30 feet or so. Since we can't see much beyond the mouth without invasive diagnostics, a quick look at the tongue can give us clues about our digestive tract functions.

Open your mouth and look at your tongue. That may sound strange, but your tongue can tell a lot about your health.

- A normal, healthy tongue is usually a pinkish, light red, with a slight white coating and is neither too thick or thin and not flabby or overlapping the teeth.
- A pale tongue can signal a vitamin or mineral deficiency and is more commonly seen among those suffering from anaemia.
- White tongue is often due to an overgrowth of candida, a fungus that causes yeast infections or oral thrush. It's actually perfectly normal for the fungus candida to live in your mouth, but when it accumulates, it can spread to the roof of the mouth, gums, tongue, tonsils and back of the throat creating white tongue, white lesions, redness and even bleeding.

- Deep cracks in the center indicate that a patient is prone to digestive issues while sores (ulcers) can indicate a deficiency.
- A patchy tongue, also called a 'geographic tongue' can reflect heat in the stomach which may manifest as acid reflux.
- A scalloped tongue (one with ridges on the outside edge) indicates fluid retention.
- A puffy tongue can suggest a lack of nutrients and moisture, while a thin tongue could suggest dehydration.

This is not an all inclusive list for a tongue diagnosis. If your tongue reading signals a problem that tracks with how your body feels, be sure to consult a holistic medical professional.

Tongue Scraping is a great way to clean up your tongue and when combined with regular Oil Pulling it can take your oral hygiene to a whole new level. It is another ancient practice that will enhance your health.

Your Eyes

- A white ring circling the iris can be indicative of both high cholesterol and arteriosclerosis, which can be symptomatic of a poor diet.
- The presence of a ring around the iris can be indicative of high blood pressure evidenced by a slow metabolism. Hypertension can lead to a host of problems if not caught early
- Environmental and food allergies and sensitivities can often present themselves as blood vessels appearing in the whites of the eyes.
- When white markings are present in the iris this may be a weakened immune system. Immune-boosting regimens

can be recommended as a way of strengthening the system so that the patient is not susceptible to illness.
- A yellowing of the white of the eye can potentially detect gallbladder and bile duct issues which can ultimately affect liver function.
- An overactive thyroid can frequently be deduced by eyes that appear to bulge slightly. This condition can cause symptoms such as fatigue, anxiety, rapid heartbeat, weight loss and trouble sleeping.
- Bags under eyes causes can be the result of a kidney problem. If your body retains fluids, bags can accumulate underneath your skin, especially when you are sleeping and not eliminating water.
- Dark circles under the eyes can be caused from lack of sleep, smoking, allergies, drinking too much alcohol and sinus infection. Dehydration is a common cause of dark circles under your eyes. When your body is not receiving the proper amount of water, the skin beneath your eyes begins to look dull and your eyes look sunken.

As you can see, it is very important for you to find out what is causing your under eye bags and dark circles. Tea bags, cucumbers, creams and surgery may treat the symptoms but they don't address the underlying problem.

Your Ears

Tinnitus: This ringing (or hissing/roaring/whooshing/buzzing/etc.) in the ears is a symptom of an underlying health condition. There are many different diseases and disorders that can cause tinnitus; these include high blood pressure, cardiovascular disease, hormonal changes, Epstein-Barr virus, Meniere's disease and tumors. Tinnitus can also cause stress, anxiety and insomnia.

Wet, sticky earwax: Some earwax is normal and beneficial; it helps prevent bacteria and other particles from entering the ear canals. But earwax with a wet and sticky texture is NOT normal and might be a sign of a mutation on the ABCC11 gene, which can increase your chances of developing breast cancer.

Red ears: Exposure to the sun or flushing from embarrassment often cause the ears to turn red. This may also occur due to hormonal changes associated with menopause or Red Ear Syndrome, a condition characterized by a burning sensation in the ears that may produce migraines and cluster headaches.

If your ears are red on a regular basis, it could be a sign of an internal health issue. Red ears may be an indicator of kidney problems.

Creased earlobes: Earlobes that contain a diagonal crease across the middle may be a sign of more probable coronary heart disease. This has been dubbed Frank's sign and occurs when tissue that surrounds the blood vessels breaks down around the ears and heart.

Indicators That You Have Some Degree of Adrenal Fatigue

What is adrenal fatigue? Very simply put, adrenal fatigue occurs when your body experiences more stress than it's able to handle. This disrupts the communication that happens between three core endocrine glands: the hypothalamus, the pituitary, and the adrenal glands themselves, and leads to dysfunction in how the adrenals function as a result.

- You're a "night person" (you have trouble getting up in the morning and you have trouble falling asleep at night, even when you're exhausted)
- Your blood pressure is either above 120/80 or below 105/70
- You get a headache after exercising
- You clench or grind your teeth
- You get dizzy when you stand up quickly
- You crave salty foods
- You perspire easily, regardless of the temperature
- You're always tired
- You need to wear sunglasses outside during the day
- You don't stay asleep at night

If two or more of these describe you, you most likely have some degree of adrenal fatigue.

What to do about it: There are many different things you can do to support your adrenals, many of which are clinical and best done with the guidance of a holistic practitioner experienced in adrenal fatigue. But first and foremost, your job is to identify all of the stressors in your life, and then one-by-one weed them out and/or drastically reduce them.

Signs of Nutrient Deficiencies

Everyone knows that we need vitamins and minerals to keep our bodies healthy. But how do you know when you aren't meeting your body's needs?

There are many telltale signs of vitamin and mineral deficiencies, the good news is that often, if you take steps to address the deficiency, the symptoms will either improve or go away altogether.

Severe Hair Loss: While everyone loses about 100 strands of hair a day, suddenly finding clumps of hair on your pillow or in your shower drain merits a mention to your doctor. It could be a sign of bigger issues, such as low iron levels, which affects your energy, or thyroid disease, which could lead to sudden unexplained weight gain or weight loss.

Always get that checked out, get a blood test to check your iron levels. If your iron levels are low, you might also always feel cold, have headaches and feel dizzy often. If you have a thyroid disorder, it can make your muscles weak, your joints ache and your skin dry and pale.

Reversing iron deficiency: The good news is you can eliminate an iron deficiency with supplements. It might take three to four months to remedy, but it is doable. Be sure to also include iron-rich foods in your diet, such as spinach and beans.

Burning Sensation in the Feet or Tongue: Talk to your doctor, who will likely order a blood test to check your B12 levels. You also might have issues with balance, constipation and dry skin.

B12 plays an essential role in your health by producing hemoglobin, part of your red blood cells that helps the cells in your body receive life-giving oxygen. The vitamin is needed for a variety of systems, like your digestive tract, to work properly.

In addition, B12 deficiency can create mild cognitive impairment, so if you're experiencing any changes in memory, thinking or behavior have your B12 level tested. Over time, B12 deficiency can permanently damage your nervous system, traveling up the spine and into the brain.

Vegans take special note: Plant-based diets eliminate most foods (meat and dairy products) rich in B12, increasing the risk of deficiency. But you can get your daily dose from almond milk, nutritional yeast, and fortified soy and coconut milk.

It can take a long time to become deficient in B12, as long as three years to deplete the liver of this important vitamin, but over time, not having enough B12 can seriously damage vital functions and it must be addressed.

Raising your B12 level: Taking B12 supplements will bring back and maintain proper B12 levels. The body does not create B12 on its own.

Healthy adults should take in 2.4 mg of B12 daily. For some, especially those with autoimmune diseases like pernicious anemia, B12 must be taken in shot form to help carry B12 directly to stomach cells.

Wounds Are Slow to Heal: If you are diligent about brushing and flossing daily and your gums are still red, swollen and bleed, you might need to boost your vitamin C intake. Another sign might be that you bruise easily.

Vitamin C is like a cement. It pulls the cells together and makes wounds heal. In fact, vitamin C has many powers, including serving as an anti-inflammatory and as an antioxidant to limit damage to cells.

Boosting vitamin C: First and foremost: If you smoke, take steps to quit. Among its many negative effects on your health, smoking limits your body's ability to absorb vitamin C. Also, eat more fruits and vegetables high in vitamin C, including kiwi, red bell peppers and, of course, oranges.

Bone Pain: If you are feeling pains in your bones, you might be deficient in vitamin D. If you're an adult and it feels like you're having growing pains like you had as a kid, tell your doctor.

Treating vitamin D deficiency: For adults, the RDA of vitamin D is 600 IU (800 IU for adults age 71 and older). Foods rich in vitamin D include salmon, herring, sardines, canned tuna, oysters, shrimp and mushrooms. Choose soy milk, orange juice, oatmeal and cereals that are fortified with vitamin D.

You can also get your daily dose by going out into the sunshine for 10 minutes without sun screen. For severe deficiencies, your doctor might prescribe a vitamin D supplement.

Unlike other vitamins and minerals, vitamin D levels are regularly tested in routine blood tests at your annual physical, so it's easy to identify deficiencies.

Irregular Heartbeat: Calcium regulates your heartbeat, so a deficiency could cause an arrhythmia, or irregular heartbeat, and even lead to chest pains.

Other signs you might not be getting enough calcium:

- Twitches around your face and mouth. Calcium works with muscles to help them contract properly.
- Muscle cramps. Without enough calcium, the muscles do not fully relax.
- Fractures. Calcium is needed for strong bones. Without it, bone loss, or osteoporosis, can lead to more fractures.

How to get more calcium: Adults should receive 1,000 mg of calcium each dayfrom food sources and supplements. Calcium-rich foods include as salmon and sardines (both of which are also excellent sources of heart-healthy omega-3 fatty acids), broccoli and bok choy.

Your Night Vision Deteriorates: If you don't take in enough vitamin A, your night vision and the sharpness of your sight could deteriorate over time. A lack of vitamin A causes the cornea to become dry and that makes the eyes cloudy and can lead to vision loss, it can also damage your retina. If you notice changes in your vision, schedule a visit with your ophthalmologist, who will examine the back of your eye.

A diet rich in vitamin A, including organic or raw milk, eggs, mangos, black-eyed peas, sweet potatoes and apricots. You can also take supplements if your diet is not meeting your needs. Aim for 700 mg of vitamin A each day and 900 mg for your man.

Simple blood tests can reveal your levels of vitamins and minerals. However, the routine blood work at your annual physical doesn't typically include most of these tests. Communicating your concerns with your primary care doctor is essential to get the tests ordered. Often the treatment for these deficiencies is fairly simple, so the key is identifying them.

Self Testing For Health Conditions

Candida / Yeast Overgrowth Test:

First thing in the morning when you wake up briefly rinse your mouth with water. Then gather some saliva in your mouth and spit it into a glass of water (be sure it is saliva and not mucus).

Keep your eye on the water for 30 minutes, especially the first few minutes. If you have yeast overgrowth you will see one or more of the following:

- Strings (legs) hanging down from the saliva
- Heavy looking saliva at the bottom of the glass
- Cloudy specks suspended in the water

If within the first 3 minutes you see strings hanging down or cloudy specks or debris sinking to the bottom of the glass, you likely have excessive overgrowth. The more you see and the faster you see it, the more candida overgrowth you have in your body.

If it takes longer than a few minutes for anything to show up, the candida is not that serious.

Iodine Patch Test:

Low levels of iodine mean your thyroid may not be functioning properly. The thyroid needs iodine to function as it helps balance hormones, regulate heartbeats, body temperature, stabilize cholesterol, maintain weight control, encourage muscle growth, keep menstrual cycles regular, provide energy, and even helps you keep a positive mental attitude.

Women are naturally prone to iodine deficiencies. That's because the thyroid gland in women is twice as large as in men, so under normal circumstances, women need more iodine. However, when women are under stress, the need for iodine can double or triple.

Two thirds of the body's iodine is found in the thyroid gland. One of the best ways to boost your iodine levels is to add sea vegetables to your diet. Just one teaspoon of sea vegetables a day can help you regain normal iodine levels. Incorporating seafood and fish into your diet can also help.

Low iodine levels can zap your energy and make you feel tired, edgy and worn out. Low iodine levels can even prevent you from getting a good night's sleep. Before you go to your doctor with complaints of tossing and turning all night, aches and pains, and just feeling "blah," you may want to perform this self-test.

Purchase a tincture of iodine. If you don't already have an iodine solution at home, you will need to purchase a tincture of iodine. These are available at most pharmacies and drug stores, as well as online.

While most iodine solutions have an orange tint, some are clear. Be sure to buy an orange solution so that it shows up on your skin. You may need to ask for it at the counter since iodine is sometimes kept behind the counter or in a glass case.

Apply the iodine in a 2 inch square on your forearm. Using a cotton swab, create a full square of iodine on your inner forearm. The square doesn't need to be precise in terms of shape or dimensions, but it should be conspicuous. If you do not want to put the iodine on your forearm, you could also put it on your abdomen or inner thigh.

Be sure to let the iodine dry for at least 20 minutes before covering it or letting it touch anything since it will stain.

Monitor the iodine for 24 hours to watch for any color fading. Check the patch every 3 or so hours to monitor how long it takes to disappear.

- If the patch is still fully visible after 24 hours, you likely don't have a deficiency.
- If the patch disappears or fades significantly over 24 hours, you may have a minor to moderate iodine deficiency.
- If the patch disappears in under 18 hours, you may have a moderate iodine deficiency.
- If the patch disappears within 4 hours you may have a severe iodine deficiency.

Iodine is rapidly eliminated from the body so high intake or toxicity is not very likely. The recommended amount of iodine is 15mg per day for maintenance and 30mg per day for treatment of an under-active thyroid.

Depending on the severity of your symptoms, you may want to consult with your doctor especially if you notice you have an enlarged thyroid.

Stomach Acid (HCL) Test:

The next time you have acid indigestion do an experiment to see if you have too much acid or not enough acid in your stomach.

- Drink 1 tablespoon of apple cider vinegar in a small amount of water.
- If after a few minutes you start to feel better and start belching; you didn't have enough acid and the vinegar raised the pH of the stomach.

- If however drinking the vinegar makes you feel worse and your stomach burns more; then you do indeed have too much acid in your stomach. Use baking soda and lemon juice in water to neutralize the acid right away.

Baking Soda-And Lemon

The alkaline power of baking soda mixed with lemon helps to neutralize acids in the digestive system. As a result, this combination soothes irritation and burning sensations. Both ingredients help with digesting heavy meals and decreasing excess gas.

Ingredients:

- 1 teaspoon of baking soda (5 g)
- juice of ½ lemon
- 1 cup of water (200 ml)

Preparation:

Mix the baking soda and lemon juice in a glass of water.
Then, stir well and wait for the blend to fizz out.

Drinking instruction:

Drink the mixture when you first notice stomach acid symptoms.

More information on stomach acid in chapter 13.

pH Acid-Alkaline Test:

If you cry and your tears burn your eyes, you are too acidic. If you pee and your urine burns, you are too acidic. If you are always tense, have no patience and easily fly off the handle, chances are you are too acidic. If you have cancer, you are too acidic.

When you are born you are alkaline, when you die you are acidic. To know what is going on in your internal environment you an purchase pH paper, it comes in a roll or individual strips which you can purchase at a pharmacy or health store.

You will quickly run the pH strip through your urine every time you pee for 2 to 3 weeks. You will learn for yourself how your body is reacting to your food and drinks. To get a true picture you want to test your urine rather than your saliva which by nature is more alkaline to prepare your food for your stomach. The urine shows what is really going on in your system. What you eat shows up in your urine's pH in about 2 hours.

- The body's pH runs from 1 to14.
- 1 you are too acidic and you are dead.
- 14 you are too alkaline and you are dead.
- A healthy reading is between 6.5 to 7.0.

If your reading is 6 or below you are too acidic and you want to force your body to become alkaline. You do this by using minerals just like the body will have to do. Eating foods high I mineral content like greens, lemons, sea vegetables and mineral supplements will force your body to be in a more alkaline state.

If your reading is too alkaline, this isn't a good thing. It means you were too acidic to begin with and your body has pulled minerals out of your bones to neutralize the blood.

Every time your urine is too acidic you will immediately choose one of the following from the list:

- green vegetable
- green salad
- green smoothie
- spirulina

- chlorophyll
- chlorella
- kelp
- fresh lemon in water
- vitamin with minerals
- mineral supplement i.e.magnesium
- capful of trace minerals
- 1 tsp baking soda in a glass of water

Depending on how acidic you are and what is causing your acidity, will depend how long it will take to force your body to stay in an alkaline state. When you are alkaline you feel better, more mellow, relaxed and laid back and you have better mental clarity. Your pH is the key to your overall health and longevity.

When you have a busy schedule and can't be thinking about alkalizing food every time you pee, an easy way to stay alkaline is to add mint flavored chlorophyll to your jug of water and drink it continually throughout the day. I take this with me when I go hiking and it keeps me hydrated and gives me more energy.

After a few weeks of testing your urine several times a day and each time forcing your body into an alkaline state, you become very aware of the difference in how you feel and you know exactly which food and drink your body doesn't like. This makes it easy to change your food choices. You also become more in tune with your body and will instinctively know when you are too acidic, without using the pH test strips.

More information about acid/alkaline balance in chapter 8.

Choosing a Holistic Doctor

Holistic medicine is a practice based on the philosophy that the human body has the natural capacity to heal itself and that symptoms of an ailment or illness are a sign that the body's built-in defenses are at work restoring health.

Holistic approaches try to find the root cause of symptoms, by looking at the whole person. Choosing a holistic-minded provider isn't always simple, however. The terminology used can be confusing. Some can serve as your primary physician, while others practice a more complementary brand of medicine and should be seen in addition to your primary doctor.

Functional Medicine Doctor:

All holistic-minded providers search for the original cause of a patient's symptoms, but certified functional-medicine doctors dig deeper than most: These physicians are MDs or DOs who specialize in solving complex health mysteries. If you are struggling with an undiagnosed problem or a collection of overlapping conditions, consider one of these doctors. (Many of the illnesses they treat are "invisible" like GI disorders, autoimmune diseases, and migraines.)

Your doc will likely work with you to create a time line of your life in order to identify any factors that may have contributed to your condition. You'll probably have lab work done too, to assess hormone and vitamin levels, and to test for things like food allergies, heavy metal overload, and genetic mutations in your DNA.

Based on all the info your physician gathers, she'll formulate a plan that will almost certainly involve dietary tweaks as nutrition plays a central role in the functional approach.

Integrative Physician:

These doctors who usually have an MD or DO practice a blend of mainstream and holistic medicine. They might prescribe an SSRI for anxiety or an antispasmodic for IBS, but they also recommend science-backed complementary therapies, such as meditation and massage, and you can expect in-depth conversations with your integrative medicine doc. She will take her time getting to know you, so she can suggest meaningful changes to your routine. Most conventional medical visits are about 15 minutes, but they usually spend around an hour with each patient.

Doctor of Osteopathy:

DOs get the same schooling as MDs, plus an extra 200 hours of training in osteopathic manipulative medicine (OMM); hands-on techniques that release tension in the muscles, joints, and nerves to promote healing. Osteopaths can treat all the same ailments as traditional docs (coughs, UTIs, ect.), but they are especially helpful for migraines, back and neck pain, period aches, arthritis, and digestive woes. There's good evidence to support OMM: In one study, people who saw a DO for migraines had less frequent attacks than people who only took meds. In another study, low-back-pain sufferers who were treated with OMM were able to take fewer painkillers.

Naturopathic Doctor:

The guiding principle of naturopathy is to encourage the body's self-healing abilities. Like an MD, a naturopathic doctor (ND) can order blood work, MRIs, and other tests, but she will recommend less-invasive treatments before drugs and surgery. Some naturopathic methods are nutrient IV infusions and homeopathic remedies. Twenty-two states offer NDs a license to practice if they've graduated from an accredited four-year naturopathic medical school. But not all of those states allow NDs to write prescriptions. So depending on your state in the U.S., if you require an Rx (say, for an inhaler or a steroid), you may also need to see an MD.

Traditional Chinese Medicine Practitioner:

Traditional Chinese Medicine (TCM) is about balancing two opposing but interdependent forces, yin and yang, and helping your vital energy, or qi, flow freely. Practitioners use many herbal and mind-body remedies, but the most well-known practice is acupuncture; the super-fine needles are thought to remove blockages along the pathways that qi travels. While a TCM practitioner shouldn't be your main doctor, acupuncture can be a potent therapy. Research shows that it helps reduce hot flashes and the frequency of migraines, and alleviates lower-back pain and osteoarthritis. A practitioner with the L.Ac degree is licensed to do acupuncture, and has a master's degree in acupuncture and Oriental medicine.

Ayurvedic Doctor:

According to the ancient Indian tradition of Ayurveda, your body's processes are governed by three life energies, or doshas: vata (space and air), pitta (fire and water), and kapha (water and earth). One of your doshas is naturally stronger than the others, but if your doshas slip too far out of balance, health issues can follow. (For example, if vata is your main dosha, you're likely full of vitality and creativity; when your vata gets too powerful, though, you may suffer from anxiety and insomnia, among other ailments.) An Ayurvedic doctor will help you restore equilibrium, using many remedies that are supported by research. For example, preliminary studies have found that active compounds in turmeric, an Ayurvedic mainstay, are just as effective as ibuprofen for knee pain from osteoarthritis. Other research has shown that breath work called pranayama can reduce anxiety, lower blood pressure, and improve sleep.

Most Ayurvedic practitioners in the U.S. don't work as primary care physicians. But, alongside your GP, they can help you manage persistent health problems, like eczema, chronic pain, or digestive distress. Narrow your search to those who completed training at a school recognized by the National Ayurvedic Medical Association.

Master Herbalist:

An herbalist is someone who specializes in handling herbs for medicinal purposes. In some cases, an herbalist focuses on growing herbs, while others may harvest or collect herbs in the wild, and some offer herbal prescriptions and advice. In many cases, an herbalist performs all three tasks, managing her own stock of herbs to ensure that they are of high quality.

An important part of herbalism is the identification of various herbs and what they can be used for. Since herbs do not have standardized ingredients like processed pharmaceuticals, an herbalist must also be skilled in collecting and storing herbs properly to ensure that they will work as intended. A professional and ethical herbalist is aware of drug interactions between various herbs and with mainstream pharmaceuticals, and she will carefully discuss a patient's situation before offering a prescription.

A competent herbalist will usually welcome the additional input of medical testing and other diagnostic tools to treat a patient's condition.

Homeopathy:

A homeopathic practitioner can be a DO, MD, naturopathic doctor, chiropractor, or acupuncturist to name a few. While some homeopathic practitioners practice homeopathy exclusively, others have professional licenses in conventional medicine and acquire further education or training to add on to their existing practices.

Homeopathy, also known as homeopathic medicine, is a

medical system that was developed in Germany more than 200 years ago. It's based on two unconventional theories:

- "Like cures like", the notion that a disease can be cured by a substance that produces similar symptoms in healthy people.
- "Law of minimum dose", the notion that the lower the dose of the medication, the greater its effectiveness. Many homeopathic products are so diluted that no molecules of the original substance remain.

Homeopathic products come from plants, minerals, or animals. Homeopathic products are often made as sugar pellets to be placed under the tongue; they may also be in other forms, such as ointments, gels, drops, creams, and tablets. Treatments are "individualized" or tailored to each person, it's common for different people with the same condition to receive different treatments. Homeopathy uses a different diagnostic system for assigning treatments to individuals and recognizes clinical patterns of signs and symptoms that are different from those of conventional medicine.

CHAPTER 7

Goddess Don't Sit Around

It's only in your thriving that you have anything to offer anyone, therefore the best investment you can ever make is in your own health.

Our bodies are meant to be active. Our ancestors had to walk, run, climb, dig and till the earth for their food. Taking care of your physical body is as important as your spiritual well-being. The Divine Feminine is a sacred energy. It does not manifest in stagnant polluted environments.

You must practice extreme self-care using real food, natural medicine, detoxification, reconnect with nature and learn how the body heals and repairs itself and keep it moving and in good physical shape, if you plan to live a long healthy life.

Find creative and accessible ways to move the energy around in your body. When your physical body doesn't get much movement or creative action, your energetic body also becomes stagnant. This can manifest as low motivation, low energy, "bad" days, or even depression and anxiety.

As soon as you feel your energy tapping into these lower vibrations, take action! The first thing you can do that will surely change the direction and release the old energy is move. Find a flow in yoga, in dance, in running/working out, or even just taking a long walk in nature.

Prolonged sitting, more than eight hours a day, increases your risk of premature death and some chronic diseases by 10-20%. Some of the health hazards from long sitting hours include:

- Cardiovascular complications; long sitting hours in the workplace leads to high blood pressure and elevated cholesterol which can increase the risk of cardiovascular complications.
- Increases risk of diabetes; when a person sits for long hours the cells in the muscles do not readily respond to the insulin produced by the pancreas. As a result, the pancreas produces more insulin which can lead to diabetes.
- Risk of muscle degeneration; a sedentary lifestyle can lead a person to developing tight hips and weak glutes.
- Leg disorders; long sitting can impact blood flow in the body causing fluid to puddle in the legs. This can lead to deep vein thrombosis.
- Increases stress level; muscles in motion trigger the release of mood enhancing hormones by supplying fresh blood and oxygen through the brain. Therefore, when a person sits for long hours their stress level increases.
- Imbalances in spinal structure; long sitting hours can lead to disc damage, inflexible spine, strained neck, sore shoulders and back.

Go Outside

Nature is healing. Get outside. Go to the park, the beach, the mountains, the water. Go for a drive, hiking, camping, fishing, picnicking. Go somewhere you enjoy and go for an aimless stroll and enjoy the sights, sounds and smells. Sit in the sunshine. Gaze at the moon and stars. Listen to the sounds of nature. Watch the birds, bees and butterflies.

When you're outdoors and your skin is exposed to the sun, it prompts your body to make vitamin D which helps your body absorb calcium, a mineral essential for bone formation.

Our ancestors spent most of their waking hours outside in nature. Too many of us spend most of our waking hours in a building of some sort rarely looking out of a window, breathing stale recycled air, under unnatural lighting.

Get Your Hands in the Dirt

Roll up your sleeves and plant a garden. Get busy digging, planting, weeding and harvesting your fresh produce. Gardening is considered a moderate intensity exercise and you can burn 300 calories in one hour of light gardening or yard work.

Dietary guidelines recommend eating at least 2 cups of vegetables and 2 cups of fruit per day to get the necessary nutrients and reduce risk of chronic disease. However, only 1 in 10 American adults meet those minimum recommendations, according to the CDC.

Gardening helps people develop a lasting habit of eating enough fruits, vegetables and herbs. Gardening also helps boost your mood and reduce stress. Gardening is a form of therapy for the body and soul.

Exposing yourself to dirt and germs can actually help you build an immune system and protect against harmful diseases later in life. You'll also get up close with some good bacteria. There are studies which say gardening and getting contact with this bacteria elevates mood and decreases anxiety.

Unbelievable as it may sound, there are some scientists who

believe playing in the mud can be as effective as antidepressants for improving your mood.

This theory is known as the "hygiene hypothesis" and claims exposure to bacteria found in your average backyard could not only boost our immune systems but help us stave off the debilitating symptoms of depression.

A lot of experts believe over cleaning and sanitizing things is actually leading people to have poor health. It sounds wrong, but think about it: if you don't ever get exposed to tiny amounts of relatively harmless bacteria, your body won't develop the tools it needs to fight off a big infection.

Planting trees helps clean the air which is particularly useful if you are living in a large town or city. On average, two mature trees produce the same amount of oxygen used by a family of four. With a big enough garden and a bit of planning, you could try to offset your family's carbon emissions through planting trees which produce lots of oxygen.

The most obvious way to save money is to create and cultivate a healthy vegetable patch. No more trips to the supermarket for expensive, and usually imported, fruits and vegetables. By concentrating on growing your own food, not only will you be eating better, more seasonal foods without the added pesticides, but you will also save cash.

Exercise

> ***"Even when all is known, the care of a man is not yet complete, because eating alone will not keep a man well; he must also take exercise. For food and exercise, while possessing opposite qualities, yet work together to produce health" Hippocrates***

- Your body stores energy in two ways, as fat and glycogen. Glycogen is the glucose stored in the muscles after eating a meal.
- Muscles store about 12 hours worth of glycogen as a ready supply.
- If you are inactive and don't use the stored energy it is turned into fat and saved to be used as energy at a later time.
- Regular exercise depletes the store of glycogen in the muscles and forces the fat cells to convert back into glycogen to use as energy.
- The magic pill everyone is looking for is activity and exercise. You don't have to be a fanatic you just have to get moving.

Daily Walks

The body is meant to move and walking is the most natural movement. Walking assists the intestines to move waste and eliminate it. Walking improves circulation and assists the heart to move blood. Walking moves the lymphatic fluids which detoxifys the body. Walking assist the lungs to expel waste through heavy breathing. If you perspire while walking you will eliminate toxins through the skin.

The body was meant to move not sit around all day. We have to move to keep or blood flowing, our digestive system moving, our bones and muscles strong. Each day, go for a brisk walk or incorporate another form of cardio into your day somehow. Grab a friend and start a walking routine together, and stick with it. Use a pedometer and try to get in 10,000 steps per day.

Walk yourself out of a bad mood in 10 minutes.

Every day walk yourself into a state of well-being and away from illness. If you walked a mile every day for a year you would have walked 365 miles, in ten years you would have walked 3650 miles. Imagine the benefits to your body, your respiratory system, your heart, your muscles, your joints and your weight, if you were to walk just one mile every day.

Walking Slows the Aging Process

We can't escape the aging process, but research suggests that we can slow it down. As we age, our body experiences a reduction in protein synthesis. This reduction leads to the development of the signs of aging, such as wrinkles.

Have you ever noticed a senior who looks decades younger than their age? This phenomenon occurs due to changes in the telomerase enzyme responsible for slowing the signs of aging. Studies suggest that physical activity may activate this enzyme, slowing the aging process in adults and seniors that exercise regularly. The telomerase enzyme is partially responsible for maintaining the integrity of DNA as well. Therefore, everything you can do to increase the activity of this enzyme will benefit you in the aging process.

Walking is the best possible exercise. Start walking today, and you can expect an increase in circulation that improves the flow of oxygen throughout the body, enhancing longevity. Stay youthful and go for a walk.

Keep Active

Find something active to do every day. Exercise for the sake of exercise is not fun and you won't stick to it. Take a dance class, dance around your house, go out dancing! Learn to play pickle ball or tennis, go biking or hiking. Take your dog for a walk, a run or throw balls and play in the park. Spend as much time outdoors as you can in the sunshine and fresh air and barefoot whenever possible.

The following are ancient exercises, spiritual and healing practices you may find interesting:

Five Tibetan Rites Exercises

Ancient Secrets of The Fountain of Youth by Peter Kelder

The 2,500-year-old Five Tibetan Rites, traditionally known as the "Fountain of Youth", is an ancient chakra-activation and energizing series of postures done in a specific sequence. This stimulates your whole glandular system boosting your metabolism among many other remarkable health benefits, like:

- Increased physical strength, flexibility and coordination
- Release from joints & back pains
- Stress relief and a steady sense of calm
- Uninterrupted, restful sleep
- Better memory, mental focus and creativity
- Improved eyesight
- Enhanced physical energy and youthfulness
- Rejuvenation of all organs
- A youthful appearance

If you're prepared to commit to an on-going practice, you'll be amazed with the results.

The exercises were reportedly created by Tibetan lamas (monks), or leaders of Tibetan Buddhism.

The Five Tibetan Exercises are so effective because they're specially designed to normalize the spinning speed of the body's seven major energy centers (chakras, or psychic vortexes).

Practitioners say youth and vigor can be achieved when these energy fields spin at the same rate. People practice the Five Tibetan Rites in order to achieve this.

When these vibrational centers are out of balance, we experience a chronic lack of energy, ill health, premature aging, an impaired endocrine system, and a sluggish metabolism.

Doing the Five Tibetan Rites regularly activates the chakras, dissolving any blocks and getting the chi energy (life energy) flowing again normally throughout every cell in your body.

As a result, your body gets rejuvenated and resumes the process of self-healing, correcting any hormonal imbalances acquired over the years due to pregnancy, dieting, a sedentary lifestyle, stress, medications, and aging.

Another important aspect of the body-mind-spirit healing effect of the Five Tibetan Rites is the focus on a specific way of breathing in between and during the exercises, coordinating the in and out breaths with certain movements.

In short, the key to the amazing power of these five Tibetan exercises is the combination of three elements:

- Daily practice
- Maintaining their correct form and sequence, and
- Synchronizing the breathing with the specific movements

The most important thing you should know is that the 5 Tibetan Rites work in conjunction with each other, so if you want to fully experience the remarkable benefits of these ancient Five Tibetan exercises it's best to do all five of them daily.

Rite 1

The purpose of the first rite is to speed up the chakras. It's common for beginners to feel dizzy during this exercise.

- Stand up straight. Stretch your arms outward until they're parallel with the floor.
- Face your palms down.

- While staying in the same spot, slowly spin your body in a clockwise direction.
- Without bending your head forward, keep your eyes open and cast toward the ground.
- Do 1 to 21 repetitions.
- Spin as many times as you can, but stop when you feel slightly dizzy. You'll be able to spin more over time. It's best to avoid excessive spinning, which is said to overstimulate the chakras.

Rite 2

During the second rite, it's important to practice deep rhythmic breathing. You should continue the same breathing pattern in between each repetition.

To do this rite, you'll need a carpeted floor or yoga mat.

- Lie flat on your back. Place your arms at your sides, palms on the floor.
- Inhale and lift your head, moving your chin toward your chest. Simultaneously raise your legs straight up, keeping your knees straight.
- Exhale and slowly lower your head and legs to the starting position. Relax all your muscles.
- Complete 1 to 21 repetitions.
- If you have difficulty straightening your knees, bend them as needed. Try to straighten them each time you perform the rite.

Rite 3

Like the second rite, the third rite requires deep rhythmic breathing. You can also practice this rite while closing your eyes, which helps you focus inward.

- Kneel on the floor, knees shoulder-width apart and hips aligned over your knees. Straighten your trunk and place your palms on the back of your thighs, below your buttocks.
- Inhale and drop your head back, arching your spine to open your chest.
- Exhale and drop your head forward, moving your chin toward your chest. Keep your hands on your thighs during the entire rite.
- Do 1 to 21 repetitions.

Rite 4

The fourth rite, sometimes called Moving Tabletop, is also done with rhythmic breathing. Your hands and heels should stay in place during the entire exercise.

- Sit on the floor and extend your legs straight ahead, feet shoulder-width apart. Put your palms on the floor at your sides, fingers facing forward. Straighten your trunk.
- Drop your chin toward your chest. Inhale and gently drop your head back.
- Simultaneously lift your hips and bend your knees until you're in a tabletop position, with your head gently tilted back. Contract your muscles and hold your breath.
- Exhale, relax your muscles, and return to starting position.
- Complete 1 to 21 repetitions.

Rite 5

The fifth rite involves both the Downward-Facing Dog and Upward-Facing Dog poses. For this reason, it's often called Two Dogs. This move also requires a steady breathing rhythm.

- Sit on the floor with your legs crossed. Plant your palms in front of you.
- Extend your feet behind you, toes curled and shoulder-width apart. Straighten your arms and arch your spine while keeping the tops of your legs on the ground. Drop your head back into Upward-Facing Dog.
- Then, inhale and lift your hips, moving your body into an upside down "V" shape.
- Move your chin toward your chest and straighten your back into Downward-Facing Dog.
- Exhale and move back into Upward-Facing Dog.
- Do 1 to 21 repetitions.
- To support your lower back, you can bend your knees when moving in between poses.

QiGong

The earliest records from the archaeological discoveries at the Ma Huang Tui Tombs revealed a series of dance like postures combined with breathing that were used for health. Researchers at the Shanghai QiGong Research Institute have theorized that QiGong probably originated from the dances of early Wu Shaman.

Dance was used in their rituals and ceremonies to induce trance states for communicating with the spirit world. Many of these dances were based upon animal movements and included the wearing of skins and masks to further heighten the effect.

In China today, QiGong is very popular. The government supports the practice of health exercises and funds research and teaching institutes. The current categories in China include a variety of systems. They are differentiated as either health exercises for preventing disease and maintaining health or for healing existing conditions of disease and recovering fully. This category also includes the use of QiGong to develop the ability to project Qi from one person to another in order to restore balance and effect healing. Specialists in QiGong develop these abilities from practitioners and they learn specific QiGong exercises for specific health problems. These have been very effective for treating chronic degenerative and stress related disorders.

The most common health maintenance systems use standing Quiescent – Dynamic postures. These can be seen in any park in China usually being practiced in the early morning. People practice in groups or individually. Often, they will stand in front of a tree or rock and they will try to absorb Qi from these natural sources of qi. The practitioner will assume a standing posture and hold a specific position for a period of time. While standing they may move their arms or body purposefully or they may hold their entire body still. Some systems use both dynamic and quiescent postures. Other systems encourage spontaneous movement of the body in accord with the flow of Qi. Generally, movement is performed standing, but there are many systems that utilize movement while seated.

Lying down postures are generally used with the very weak, elderly or ill persons and tend primarily to focus on breathing and visualization methods.

In any of the circumstances, the primary goals are to activate the Qi and increase the circulation of Qi through the channels and internal organs of the entire body. This is the basic approach to the QiGong Systems in general. Any system may utilize any number of specific variations in accomplishing this goal.

Tai Chi

Tai Chi (pronounced "tie chee") is an ancient Chinese therapy that connects the mind, body, and spirit through a series of slow, gentle, flowing postures that create a kind of synchronized dance, based on th martial arts. This is great gentle stretching, breathing, and meditation in motion. Tai Chi may be done in flat shoes or barefoot.

Practicing tai chi can improve both your physical and mental health. This safe and gentle form of exercise is appropriate for all ages and fitness levels. Plus, it is easily adaptable to certain physical limitations and health conditions.

To get started, look for tai chi classes taught by experienced instructors at senior centers, health clubs, and fitness studios.

Yoga

Yoga's time line coincides with our own 'cradle of civilization', which began in the Tigris and Euphrates Valley of Mesopotamia, more than 5000 years ago. In Northern India around the same time, a civilization was already developed in the Indus Valley, rich in art, jewelry, and cultural artefacts, including some forms of writing. Agriculturally minded, they specialized in growing wheat and barley.

While Yoga has amazing benefits and adds to a longer life, the true history and philosophy of Yoga is rooted in the spiritual, and not just the physical. Most yoga practitioners do believe in a divine being or deities. Yoga is about self-awareness and discovering the divine within, creating a strong sense of self and of humankind.

Through the many different styles of yoga, you'll notice a common, consistent theme: self-healing. Whether you choose to practice Yin or prefer Vinyasa, practicing any style of yoga gives you the opportunity to turn inward and learn more about yourself so that you can be of greater service to the people and the world around you. If you're new, it's worth trying different styles to find which best resonates with you.

CHAPTER 8

Acid—Alkaline Balance

"Every single person who has cancer has a pH that is too high. Cancer does not survive in an alkaline state". Dr Otto Warburg

Acidity

When we are born we are alkaline. When we die we are acidic. Acid/Alkaline balance is vital for keeping your body healthy and long living. In our daily life we don't put enough attention to it.

What is acid/alkaline balance? Acid/alkaline balance is the pH of the body's fluids, tissues and blood. pH stands for potential of Hydrogen, which is a measure of the acidity or alkalinity of a solution, such as a mixture of liquids.

Over acidity can become a dangerous condition that weakens all body systems. Acidic blood pH levels lead to many deadly diseases such as cancer, heart disease, and death.

Acid environment around the cells also causes stress and a build-up of waste products that clog the lymph system and make it harder to move the waste out of the body. This build-up of waste in your tissues is the basis of disease. Over time even mild acidity in your body can cause problems such as:

- Premature aging
- Frequent headaches, sinusitis
- Constipation, hemorrhoids
- Weight gain, obesity
- Diabetes and insulin disorders
- Osteoporosis, hip fractures
- Osteoarthritis, joint pain, aching muscles
- Hormonal imbalance
- Liver, Bladder and Kidney conditions, including kidneys and gallstones
- Weakened Immune system
- High blood pressure, increased stress
- Low energy and chronic fatigue
- Neurological Diseases: MS, ALS, Parkinson's, Alzheimer's
- Cystic Fibrosis
- Cardiovascular damage, including the constriction of blood vessels, clogged arteries, weakened veins, and the reduction of oxygen
- Fibromyalgia
- Acid indigestion and flatulence
- Lymphatic congestion
- Yeast, fungal overgrowth.

Acidification of the body comes as a result of three things:

1. Eating too many acidifying foods and drinks which create an acid ash in your body.
2. Bacteria, yeast, fungi not only create acidic toxins in your body, they also proliferate in an acidic body and further acidify your body.

3. Lack of proper alkaline buffers such as certain minerals that neutralize acids.

With a proper diet and intake of alkaline-mineral rich food, water and alkaline supplements when needed, you will replenish your body's capacity to neutralize excess acids. By eating 80% alkalizing foods and only 20% acidic foods you'll eliminate the production of excess acid in your body. Food is the cause and food is the cure of most disease.

What Should My pH Levels Be?

The pH value is a measure of how acidic or alkaline something is, and ranges from 0 to 14. Anything ranging from 0 to 6 is considered acidic, 7 is neutral, and 8 to 14 is alkaline, or basic. However, the pH value in people's bodies varies greatly throughout the body. Some parts are alkaline and other parts are acidic. The stomach, for example, has hydrochloric acid in it, making it highly acidic, but this is an important digestive necessity in order to break down food. Blood, however, is always slightly alkaline, and it is extremely serious and sometimes fatal if it becomes acidic. This is why it's important to eat foods that support an alkaline environment in the body.

How Do I Check My pH?

pH strips are relatively inexpensive and can be found in pharmacies, health stores and online. They give a fast and accurate reading of your body's acidity and alkaline levels. These strips give you a convenient method to monitor your pH levels in the privacy of your home or anywhere you are. They are small and easily fit in your pocket or purse.

You can use either saliva or urine to test your pH. Results

appear 15 seconds after your test is administered, and the strips come with an easy-to-read chart to see what range you are in. I prefer checking the urine which is the end fluid that has traveled throughout your body giving you a truer reading of your body's pH. Saliva is naturally more alkaline and any traces of food or drink affect the reading.

To get a clear picture of how your body processes your food and drink do this two week test.

Two Week Test:

1. Testing your pH first thing in the morning before eating, drinking or brushing your teeth, this is important. Your body naturally detoxifies during your sleep so the reading may be a little acidic.
2. Test your urine Every Time you pee throughout the day, this reading will be a reflection of what you ate and drank 2 hours earlier. This will let you know if your body likes what you are putting in it or not.

Everytime you are too acidic do one of the following to quickly bring your body back to an alkaline state:

- Eat a green salad
- Drink a green smoothie
- Drink a shot of wheatgrass
- Take a dose of chlorophyll
- Take a mineral supplement
- Drink a glass of lemon water
- Add a teaspoon of baking soda to a glass of water
- Drink alkaline water

After doing this several times day for 2 weeks you will learn what you should and should not eat. You will begin to feel the difference in how you feel when you are alkaline and acidic. When you are alkaline you feel more calm, easy going, laid back. When you are acidic you are short tempered, uptight, irritable, on edge. This two week test is an amazing eye opener and will change the way you eat. It's like getting a peek into your internal environment without a doctor or lab test.

In the future you rarely need the pH strips because you will know you are acidic just by how you feel, and you will know how to quickly return to an alkaline balance.

How Do I Keep My Body Alkaline?

The only thing that alkalizes the body is minerals. The only place there are minerals are in rocks and broken down rocks in soil. We get minerals from the plants which send their roots down into the soil to pull the minerals up into the plant. You have to eat plants to get minerals and stay alkaline. End of story.

Electric foods are alkaline foods which helps the body to heal and nourish itself. Alkaline foods have a pH of 7.0 and above. Electric foods are found in nature. They are not hybrid, genetically modified, and they are non-irradiated.

Chlorophyll

Chlorophyll is the green blood of the plant which is very alkaline, the greener the plant the better. Chlorophyll is very much like our blood and helps us to make better blood in our bodies. There have been successful emergency blood transfusions using chlorophyll.

You'll want to start by incorporating more fruits, vegetables, leafy greens and fresh herbs into your diet .The nutrients and minerals in these alkaline foods will help get rid of inflammation and toxins which contribute to acidosis. Getting rid of soft drinks, refined sugar, processed foods, limiting coffee, alcohol and excessive amounts of meat will allow your body to become more alkaline.

How does the body alkalize itself?

Exercise helps your body sustain and restore its neutral pH balance of tissues, as well as blood and cellular fluids. Doing aerobic exercise is the best way to maintain the acid-alkaline equilibrium in your body because it works your muscles and can help reduce the accumulation of acid in your system.

The largest store of minerals in your body is in your bones. When your body is too acidic it will pull the calcium and minerals out of your bones to keep your blood alkaline so you don't die. This of course will cause weak bones, fractures, back aches, osteopenia and osteoporosis. All of which can be reversed by changing your diet, remaining alkaline and doing resistance exercises.

Acidic Foods

- Sugar
- Dairy
- Meat, processed meat
- Processed food
- Carbonated beverages, energy drinks
- Coffee
- Alcohol

You can find food charts in books and online. Not all acidic foods are bad for you but we eat too many of them. The rule of thumb is to eat 80% alkaline foods and 20% acidic foods. Pick and choose whatever you like just stay in that ratio and check our pH often until you figure out what works for you.

What Does "alkaline forming" Foods Mean?

This means that while a food might not be alkaline in nature, when broken down by the body is produces an alkaline effect. One example is that citrus fruits like grapefruits and lemons, while containing citric acid, are actually alkalizing once you eat them.

CHAPTER 9

Glowing Goddess Skin

Beautiful skin requires commitment, not a miracle.

Skin problems are the number one reason for people going to the doctor. The skin is the mirror of internal health. Skin disorders can be physically and emotionally daunting as a glowing skin is an important aspect of physical beauty. Various skin conditions can leave us feeling embarrassed and uncomfortable.

Our skin is a reflection of our overall health, which is why glowing, beautiful skin often results from proper care, hydration and eating a nutrient-dense diet. On the other hand, skin ridden with whiteheads, blackheads and other types of pimples can indicate oxidative damage, poor nutrition, digestion and hormone imbalances.

Once believed to strike most often during teen years, acne is now affecting millions of adult women, many of which never had a problem with acne in the past. Some women will only deal with acne during puberty and their teenage years, but others will suffer well into adulthood, especially during times of stress and hormonal changes. While acne among adult women is usually linked to hormonal shifts and imbalances that occur during the menstrual cycle, or when transitioning into menopause, it's important to consider elevated stress levels, a lack of sleep and a poor diet might also be root causes.

A major indicator of healthy skin is a natural glow. But factors like stressful lifestyles, hectic work schedules, inadequate sleep, lack of nutritional diet, pollution, excess sun rays, excessive smoking, and drinking alcohol can make your skin dull and dry . All of these are part and parcel of your life, and some you cannot run away from. While you cannot hold on to your age, you can surely slow down the loss of glow and radiance from your skin.

Eat a Healthy Diet

Too much sugar or too much alcohol will rob you of your divine feminine radiance reserves. So even if you're young, remember beauty does have a short shelf life. My recommendation is to use ingredients that are unrefined, organic, pastured raised, and properly prepared. Alter your recipes to exclude refined sugar, white flour, processed salt and unhealthy fats. Signs of aging can be slowed by the magical phytonutrients, vitamin C, and high water content that they contain. The high water content will hydrate your skin preventing wrinkles and the vitamin C and phytonutrients protect against cell damage.

Healthy proteins and nutritious fruits and vegetables go a long way toward making skin glow. Add these elements to your diet to see quick results:

- Omega 3 fatty acids. These are found in fish and walnuts, and are especially beneficial to your skin.
- Vitamin C. This will help existing pimples heal faster, so eating a few servings of citrus fruits and spinach will help. Vitamin C stimulates collagen synthesis and

protects against wrinkles. So stock up on kiwi, oranges, and grapefruit, which are all rich in the nutrient.

- Fiber-rich foods. Fresh vegetables, nuts, and unprocessed fruit helps keep a fine balance and to be regular, not sluggish, in the gastrointestinal area. You may look and feel tired and sickly and have headaches and abdominal complaints, if you do not have regular bowel movements once or more every day.
- Eat antioxidant-rich Food. Load up on grapes, berries and nuts like pecans and walnuts, which are rich in polyphenols such as ellagic acid and resveratrol. Research has linked this type of antioxidant combats free radicals to help protect skin cells from UV damage like hyper pigmentation.
- Minerals are magic. Zinc, copper and selenium are required for collagen production, a healthy immune system and keeping your skin elastic. Add more of these minerals to your diet with foods like chicken, lean beef, walnuts, chickpeas, and dried fruits.
- Aim to drink 6 to 8 glasses of water a day. You have to hydrate your skin from the inside out. Also the water will clear your skin and make it glow because it makes it easier for your body to flush out toxins quickly. Water bottles, as with straws, the constant pursing creates lines and aggravates existing ones around the mouth. Sip filtered water from a glass at home, and carry a reusable bottle with a spout so that you can squirt it into your mouth instead of sucking on the top.
- Eat less sugar and salt. Try to consume less than 45g of sugar on a daily basis, and cut down on salty foods. Proteins in your skin react with excessive sugar, which causes your skin to wrinkle and age faster. Eating too much salt can make your face look bloated. Excess sodium

in your diet can suck the moisture out of skin and leave it dull and dry.

- Kick The Caffeine. Can't figure out why you have dry skin? Caffeine may be the culprit. Replace the java with H2O, and add fruit slices, like orange or lemon, to enhance the flavor.
- One less serving of alcohol per day can make a noticeable difference in your appearance. Alcohol dehydrates the skin which causes wrinkles while inflaming tissue. Combat these effects by watering down wine and liquor with club soda and drinking a glass of water between alcoholic beverages.
- Foods like salmon, herring, and trout provide our skin with oils that lubricate cells and reduce inflammation. They are also heavy in omega-3 fatty acids, which play a key role in keeping our skin smooth.

Supplemental Skin Savers

A healthy glow starts on the inside, so get a head start by taking a daily multivitamin with C or E to combat fine lines and pesky wrinkles. For smooth skin, stock up on fatty acids like omega-3 and omega-6.

Research has shown that taking certain vitamins and other nutritional supplements, including vitamin D, fish oil, collagen, and vitamin C, may help improve skin hydration and help keep your skin healthy and nourished.

Exfoliate Your Skin

One of the best ways to brighten skin and boost its glow both immediately and long term is by exfoliating. The process removes skin's outer layer of dead cells so its surface is smoother and clearer and reflects light.

Exfoliate Everywhere. Although often overlooked, our neck, chest, and hands get plenty of sun exposure. Give these body parts some extra TLC by exfoliating them regularly to reveal fresh, bright skin.

Dry Skin Brushing

Increase your circulation and give your body some extra exfoliation by using a dry brush once a week for bright and smooth skin. Afterwards, apply a creamy lotion or oil to prevent flakes and seal in moisture. Exfoliate - Shower - Moisturize.

Cleanse Regularly

Key to luminous skin: clearing your "canvas" by thoroughly removing debris like dirt, oil and pollution particles that can clog pores and cause dullness. Wash your face morning and night by massaging in a small dollop of face cleanser lightly with fingers in circular motions, working from the inside of the face out for full coverage.

Over-washing your face removes natural oils which can actually cause your face to over-produce oil. It's only necessary to wash your face twice a day, once in the morning and once at night. If you have dry skin, wash at night, but just rinse with cold water when you get up.

Hydrate

Lack of hydration makes your complexion dull and even accentuates wrinkles. Apply a topical moisturizer morning and evening to replenish hydration.

Ice Treatment

Chill out. Run ice cubes over your face until they melt. Your pores love this skin shocker.

Witch Hazel

Witch hazel is a natural skin-tightening astringent and can be used to deflate under-eye bags. Soak two cotton pads in cold witch hazel and apply one to each closed eye for five minutes.

Hang Upside Down

Use an inversion table or bend over. Hanging your head upside down for three minutes a day is a long-term strategy for getting that lit-from-within glow.

Stay Active

Exercise gives your face a healthy glow by increasing blood flow. And when you sweat, it clears the body of toxins and removes dead skins cells so new ones can grow. Without regular exercise you may see an increase in age spots, so grab your dancing shoes and get to work.

Get Plenty of Sleep

Not getting enough sleep can cause stress, which leads to breakouts and a dull complexion. Bottom line: Don't deprive your body and skin of sleep, it uses that time to regenerate and recover from your day-to-day activities.

The best way to avoid sleep lines is to sleep on your back.

Sleeping in certain positions may result in sleep lines, after a while, these lines can turn into deep-set wrinkles. Use smooth pillowcases, satin or silk is best, or buy the softest, highest-thread-count fabric you can. In order to keep skin healthy, make sure you change your pillowcase at least once every two weeks.

Wear Sunglasses

Squinting in the sun can contribute to crow's feet.

No Tanning Beds

"Avoid the tanning bed at all costs," says DermaDoctor founder Dr. Audrey Kunin. "Even being at the beach without sunscreen is better than a tanning bed.

Opt for Oil

Want silk-like skin, fast? After a shower, while your skin's still damp, apply olive oil all over your body and pat dry with a damp towel.

Love Your Lips

Your lips lack the same amount of melanin found in the rest of your skin, so there is less natural protection against the environmental elements. Apply moisture hydrating balms regularly.

Treat Your Feet

Get smoother feet in a flash with a mixture of salt and lotion, or by rubbing them with olive oil. Rinse thoroughly, and push back the cuticles as you towel dry.

Manage Stress

Uncontrolled stress can make your skin more sensitive and trigger acne breakouts and other skin problems. To encourage healthy skin and a healthy state of mind take steps to manage your stress. Get enough sleep, set reasonable limits, scale back your to-do list and make time to do the things you enjoy. The results might be more dramatic than you expect.

Treat Your Divine Self

Whether it's a facial, massage, or even a pedicure, be sure to pamper yourself. Your health and appearance are positively influenced by increasing your emotional and mental well-being. A visit to the spa is a foolproof way to promote stress relief and relaxation.

CHAPTER 10

Goddess Breath

No self-respecting Goddess can have bad breath.

Bad breath is a problem that can be caused by anything from an overload of bacteria in your mouth, underlying dental problems, or just a stinky snack with foods like garlic or onions. But that mouthwash you buy at the store; why is it electric green or bright purple? If you take a moment to read the label, you'll find you're not getting much more than a mouthful of chemicals, artificial coloring, and flavoring that does little to help your breath for more than a half hour or so. It may actually do more damage long-term as one of the most popular ingredients in mouthwash is ethyl alcohol, which can weaken the lining of your gums. Although inconclusive, Stanford University has conducted research that may link certain mouthwash to oral cancer. So the next time you need to freshen your breath, buy or make your own natural mouthwash and toothpaste. It's inexpensive, refreshing, effective and healthy.

Oral Health in Ancient Times vs Modern Times

Most of the world's population, especially indigenous cultures and developing countries, still use old-world techniques to keep their teeth clean, if they use anything at all.

But are modern oral hygiene products and techniques infinitely better than the sticks, animal bristles and bones, twigs, feathers and porcupine quills that non-first-world societies used centuries ago, or continue to use today to clean their teeth?

Is what one eats more important in determining oral hygiene than the materials used to clean the teeth and gums?

Sally Fallon, president of the Weston A. Price Foundation, a nonprofit nutrition education foundation, tells Mother Nature Network that in traditional societies that have no access to Western foods with processed sugars and white flour, many of these indigenous people have no cavities, and flash smiles with perfect pearly white teeth, even though tooth brushing is rare, (or was rare, depending on the society). "Within a very short time of forgoing their traditional, native diets, though, cavities become evident," says Fallon, adding that the next generation of natives who eat processed food will begin to develop crooked teeth.

Fallon points to the research pioneered by the foundation's namesake, Dr. Weston Price, an Ohio dentist. The late Price, in the 1930s, traveled the world as a sort of a cultural dental anthropologist. His book, "Nutrition and Physical Degeneration," features many photos of the teeth of various native societies, from isolated villagers in the Swiss Alps, to the Maori of New Zealand, to the cold water fishermen of Scotland's Hebrides islands.

Price discovered a substance he termed "Activator X" that all the natives with healthy teeth had in their saliva. Price didn't know exactly what Activator X was, but shortly after his studies, science classified the cavity combating compound as vitamin K. A study published in the Journal of Dental Research states that in 1942, it was proven that vitamin K prevented the formation of acid buildup, which is a major cause of cavities.

Some of the foods that are high in vitamin K that Price observed traditional societies consuming were:

- Chicken or goose liver
- Fermented foods like sauerkraut
- Grass-fed animal fat
- Grass-fed, raw butter
- Egg yolks

Other foods high in vitamin K are:

- Kale and leafy greens
- Natto
- Brussels Sprouts
- Broccoli
- Cabbage
- Scallions
- Prunes
- Fermented dairy
- Asparagus
- Basil
- Soybeans
- Cucumber
- Extra Virgin Olive Oil

Bad Breath

Bad breath can be embarrassing and in some cases may even cause anxiety. It's no wonder that store shelves are overflowing with gum, mints, mouthwashes and other products designed to fight bad breath.

The following products are only temporary measures because they don't address the cause of the problem but while you are working on the underlying cause these may help:

- Try serving fresh parsley on your plate. Chewing on parsley can help freshen breath and eliminate odors caused by food.
- Breath mints with xylitol help kill bacteria while freshening breath.
- Drink plenty of water throughout the day to help prevent dry mouth.
- Clicking your molars together several times creates more saliva in your mouth. You need saliva to kill bacteria.

Gum Disease

Gum disease affects more than half of all Americans over 30 years old. Even with a daily oral hygiene routine in place, gum disease, also known as periodontal disease or periodontitis, can find its way into your busy lives. Periodontal disease is the result of advanced gingivitis, which is caused by a buildup of bacteria. Once your gums become irritated and infected by the bacteria, periodontal disease can cause pockets to form as the gums pull away from your teeth.

Although there are some invasive dental procedures and treatments specific to gum disease available, there are natural remedies that you can implement at home in your daily routines to improve your oral health and maybe even reverse the symptoms of periodontal disease. If you are missing teeth and require dental implants or tooth replacements of any kind your dentist needs to make sure your gums are healthy and strong enough to handle it.

Eat Healthy Food, Avoid Junk Food

Eat lots of fruits and vegetables, especially those that are rich in nutrients like vitamin C. This vitamin is basic to the health of your gums. Vitamin C helps to prevent gum problems, prevents oral diseases and advances gum recovery. In this way, have lots of oranges, strawberries, pineapples, prunes and vegetables like broccoli, cauliflower, asparagus, carrots, etc. Avoid sugary foods and beverages. They are ideal for the growth of bacteria.

Water for Oral Health

One final piece to the puzzle is to drink plenty of water. One of the top ways to fight bacteria in your mouth is to keep it from becoming dry, allowing saliva to do its part in naturally protecting your mouth. Occasionally rinsing with water is also beneficial in removing grime and preventing buildup.

More tips for preventing and reversing receding gums:

- Maintain a proper oral hygiene.
- Use a soft bristle brush for cleaning your teeth.
- Use tender and roundabout strokes while brushing.
- Brush along your gum lines and never push your gums in an upward direction.
- Don't use too substantial a toothbrush. A brush having a small head and soft brush is ideal for your mouth.
- Don't forget to floss as it is essential for uprooting plaque.
- The ideal condition is to brush and floss after every supper. On the off chance that, however, it is not conceivable every time, at least flush your mouth properly with water after dinners.

Natural Oral Health Treatments

Oil Pulling

One effective method to improving your breath, gum disease and reversing periodontitis is oil pulling. Many individuals have implemented coconut oil into their daily regimen. Thanks to its mild, sweet flavor, coconut oil is preferred as a natural mouthwash over other traditional oils such as sunflower or sesame oil. Another great reason to use coconut oil is that you can warm it into a liquid that is perfect for pulling out the dirt, food particles, toxins, and other bacteria out of your mouth and ultimately improving the symptoms you experience from periodontitis.

It is believed that this traditional Ayurvedic technique, also provides relief from headaches, constipation, candida infections, congestion, cold sores, joint pains, and various other ailments. It needs to be followed first thing in the morning, on an empty stomach before you even brush your teeth.

- Swish one tablespoon of sesame oil, sunflower oil, olive oil, or coconut oil in your mouth like a mouthwash for 15 to 20 minutes, until the oil becomes thinner and turns milky and foamy.
- Spit it out in a trash can (not your sink as it can clog the drain) and then rinse your mouth with water.
- It should be followed by tooth brushing and rinsing of the mouth.
- Do this daily at least for 15 days up to a month to see encouraging results.
- Warning: Do not gargle or swallow the oil as it contains bacteria and toxins.
- You should use this method at least once per day, more often if you have advanced gum disease, and over a very

short time you will notice healthier gums, less bleeding and maybe even reverse receding.

Oil pulling is an ancient Ayurvedic health practice that has been used for thousands of years.

Tongue Scraping

Tongue scraping is another ancient Ayurvedic health practice the Divine Feminine used. Ancient writings say that by cleaning the tongue, this removes foul smell, tastelessness and by taking out dirt coated on the tongue, teeth and mouth brings relish immediately. No doubt, people who clean their tongue on a daily basis can validate the invigorating effects this practice has.

There are many benefits to this daily practice as far as oral health, and overall physical, mental, and spiritual health. Since the oral cavity is one of the main gateways between your mind/body and the environment, maintaining the health of this connection is critical to general well-being.

Tongue scraping should be performed on a daily basis. This ancient practice helps to stimulate the internal organs through energetic connections with the rest of the body, improve digestion by increasing your sense of taste, and cleanse the body by removing bacteria from your oral cavity.

- The tongue should be gently scraped from back to front for 7 to 14 strokes.
- The scraper may be rinsed off between strokes if there is a lot of accumulation.
- Some people report stimulation of the gag reflex during scraping, which may indicate that the scraping is too aggressive. If this occurs with gentle scraping, begin slightly more forward on the tongue to avoid the gagging reflex.

Essential Oils for a Healthy Mouth

Essential oils are extremely beneficial for the teeth and gums. According to the Journal of International Oral Health, essential oils can inhibit plaque, remove stains, eliminate the bacteria, and keep the teeth and gums healthy.

A few drops of these oils can be added to your DIY toothpaste, tooth powders, mouthwash and whiteners. Take care to never directly apply essential oil to your skin or mouth or take it internally without diluting it with a carrier oil as they are very concentrated and some can burn and cause irritation.

Tea Tree Oil: The tea tree oil is packed with antibacterial, antifungal, antiviral and antiprotozoal properties. Therefore, this essential oil reduces bacterial load and yeast and fungal infections and relieves the symptoms of gingivitis. Moreover, it eliminates bad breath and maintains the oral health.

Clove Oil: Clove oil contains eugenol, which is used for its anesthetic and analgesic action in dentistry. Clove essential oil could easily be the strongest, most powerful essential oil for bad breath. It has potent antiviral, antibacterial, antimicrobial, antiseptic, and antifungal properties. While masking and eventually getting rid of the bad breath, clove essential oil will treat toothaches. How? It has numbing effects.

Cinnamon Essential Oil: Cinnamon oil has been found to have a lot of health benefits. It has antibacterial and antifungal properties that make it helpful for gum disease.

It has also been hailed for its ability to fight Strep mutans, the bacteria that cause tooth decay and gum infections.

Myrrh Essential Oil: Myrrh has antiseptic and soothing properties. So it works well for mouth ulcers and for soothing inflamed gums. Myrrh essential oil also helps to improve blood flow, thus helping to support gum tissue and improve oral health. May also help with receding gums.

Spearmint Essential Oil: This is similar to peppermint essential oil. Spearmint acts as an antiseptic and kills germs in the mouth. It also has soothing and healing properties that are helpful for mouth ulcers and gum inflammation.

Other essential oils for oral health:

- peppermint
- eucalyptus
- lemon
- wintergreen
- rosemary
- thyme

To use of the oil, add a few drops (1 or 2) of the oil to your toothbrush and use it to brush your teeth, gums, and tongue. When done brushing, rinse your mouth thoroughly with clean water.

Do not swallow the essential oil. Though effective in eliminating the repugnant smell, you should never swallow it. The active components in essential oils are too powerful and can be unsafe if ingested.

Be careful with the hot essential oils like cinnamon, clove or thyme as they may burn your mouth. You can add a drop to your toothpaste to dilute it a bit.

Use 100 percent pure therapeutic essential oils not aromatherapy oils.

Essential Oil Mouth Rinse Recipe

Ingredients:

- Add 1 tbsp. of sea salt to 2 cups of warm water and mix let it cool.
- Add 3 drops each of peppermint, Tea tree, Cinnamon, myrrh EOs
- and 1 drop of clove
- and a few drops of carrier oil.

Use to rinse your mouth (for 30 seconds) twice a day.

Mineralizing Tooth Powder Recipe

Ingredients:

- 4 parts bentonite clay
- 1 part baking soda
- 1/2 part myrrh gum powder
- 1/2 part ground cloves
- 1/2 part ground stevia
- essential oils of cloves and cinnamon

Directions:

1. Add all ingredients to a mason jar. Tightly close the lid and shake jar until well combined.
2. To use, apply a small amount of tooth powder to your tooth brush with a spoon and brush as you normally would.

Note: For a minty variation substitute peppermint leaf powder for the ground cloves and peppermint essential oils for the essential oils of cloves and cinnamon.

Natural Teeth Whiteners

We don't need any unhealthy, crazy chemicals to keep our Goddess teeth white. Nor do we need to drop major money on expensive teeth whitening products. We can easily make our own natural teeth whitening paste at home with just a few simple ingredients. There are many recipes, the following is an easy one to try.

This paste is made with just 3 ingredients, two of which are well-known for their teeth whitening benefits; in fact, many whitening toothpastes, mouth washes, whitening strips, contain one or both of them.

Baking soda: Baking soda teeth whitening pastes are tried-and-true. A number of studies have found that toothpaste with baking soda whitens teeth more effectively than toothpastes without baking soda.

Not only does baking soda gently polish away stains on teeth, but studies have found that it also helps kill unhealthy bacteria and prevent plaque build-up by creating an alkaline environment in your mouth (a very big bonus!).

Hydrogen peroxide: Hydrogen peroxide teeth whitening strips and mouthwashes are also popular and for good reason: peroxide is a natural bleaching agent and helps to improve gum health by keeping unhealthy bacteria under control.

Peppermint essential oil: Not only does peppermint essential oil provide flavor and freshen breath, but it also helps fight bacteria. No, it doesn't help whiten teeth so if you don't have or like it, you can leave it out or use any other essential oil you prefer.

Teeth Whitening Recipe

Ingredients:

- 1 tsp aluminum-free baking soda
- 2 tsp 3% food grade hydrogen peroxide
- 1 drop peppermint essential oil

*Food grade hydrogen peroxide differs greatly from the run-of-the-mill hydrogen peroxide found in the drugstore, which is not safe to ingest as it contains many heavy metals.

Directions:

- Mix the baking soda, hydrogen peroxide, and essential oil into a smooth paste.
- Dip your toothbrush in the paste and brush *gently* for about 2 minutes before brushing with regular toothpaste.
- Use no more than once a week, since baking soda is abrasive and you don't want to damage your enamel!

CHAPTER 11

Goddess Bones

"To thrive in life you need three bones. A wish bone. A back bone. And a funny bone." Reba McEntire

Good bone health really does have a lot to do with a healthy diet. Eat fresh, whole foods and make your meals from scratch. It's not always easy, but you'll be better for it.

In fact, loading up on produce is one of the best ways to improve bone density. Make a habit of eating six to nine daily servings of fruits and vegetables. It's time to acquire a taste for Brussels sprouts, turnip, and mustard greens! You'll keep your blood alkaline and benefit from other bone-friendly nutrients in these foods like phosphorous and vitamin K.

How about dried plums? They're good for more than keeping you regular. A 2011 study in the British Medical Journal revealed that women who consumed 8 to 10 prunes a day had higher bone mineral density than those who ate dried apples. Why prunes? They give you potassium and boron, both good for bone health.

Strontium for bone health is another important nutrient. The main food source for strontium is seafood, so treat yourself to shrimp, clams, crab, and lobster. If you're not a seafood person, other sources include wheat bran, poultry, and root vegetables like sweet potatoes.

Prevent and Reverse Osteoporosis

Knowing the real cause of bone loss and brittle bones is your first step to understanding how to prevent it. Taking care of your health means addressing nutritional deficiencies, getting plenty of exercise, and taking in the essential nutrients your body needs.

In our society people drink coffee, soda, alcohol and eat fast, processed foods high in bad fats, protein, sugar, flour and salt like there is no tomorrow. This creates not only a nutrient deficient body, but also an acidic one at that.

Bones are largely made up of calcium and phosphorus and also use a variety of other nutrients to form properly. An acidic state in the body needs a buffer to keep things in balance and prevent us from literally dying. The most common buffer your body uses, is the precious alkaline calcium that it finds in your bones.

So if you are concerned about losing bone mass, before you consider any pharmaceutical pill or supplement, go to the source and stop pulling calcium from your bones unnecessarily. Clean up your diet first and foremost, as there lies the power to build and repair anything and everything in your body properly.

Risk factors for Osteopenia and Osteoporosis:

- High sugar intake
- Cigarette smoking
- Excessive alcohol and caffeine intake
- High-animal-protein diets (encourage mineral loss in the urine)
- Low-calorie weight loss diets

- High milk and dairy product consumption
- Drinking exclusively distilled water
- Physical inactivity
- Excessive physical exercise
- Never having been pregnant
- Diuretics (water pills)
- Anti-seizure medications
- Anticoagulants ('blood thinners')
- Antacid abuse, all anti-ulcer drugs
- Digestive disorders leading to malabsorption of trace minerals
- Overactive endocrine glands (especially hyperthyroidism)
- Long-term use of prescription steroids like prednisone
- Numerous vitamin and mineral deficiencies

One of the easiest and best steps to preventing unnecessary bone loss is cutting the junk out of your diet. This means trading in your soda, boxed food, canned food, and fast food for nutrient-rich whole food. A whole-food diet consists of organic fruits and vegetables, nuts, seeds, whole grains, wild-caught fish, lean protein and healthy fats.

There are several ways to reverse osteoporosis naturally and diet, healthy lifestyle and nutritional supplementation all help.

NO Carbonated Beverages

Cutting down on carbonated beverages is one of the most important ways to reverse osteoporosis naturally. These drinks drain valuable calcium from the bones and make them weak. Research has shown that women falling within the age group of 16 to 20 years already display signs of bone loss due to their high intake of soft drinks. These carbonated beverages also contain high amounts of phosphates, which further causes calcium loss in the body.

Cut Out Sugar

Diet is an important part of a healthy lifestyle and cutting down on sugars is necessary to reverse osteoporosis naturally. Since refined sugar contains virtually no vitamins or minerals at all, it dilutes our nutrient intake. This results in an across-the-board 19% reduction in all vitamins and minerals in our diet. Thus, we are getting less magnesium, folic acid, vitamin B6, zinc, copper, manganese, and other nutrients that play a role in maintaining healthy bones.

Beware of Dairy

Interestingly, those foods most often recommended for healthy bones (milk and dairy products) are actually high in phosphorus and may therefore promote osteoporosis. In fact, the more dairy products consumed, the worse the incidence of osteoporosis. (In areas of the world where dairy product consumption is the lowest, osteoporosis is virtually non-existent.)

Raw milk is alkaline and nutritious with live enzymes to help digest it. Pasturized homogenized milk is acidic, has no enzymes, and is more harmful than helpful.

Eat More Fiber

Sugar and insulin levels can be lowered by increasing fiber intake. If you eat a lousy meal fiber supplements consumed just before the meal aid in slowing down sugar and fat absorption in the body. This further helps in reducing the cholesterol and blood sugar levels in the body to a great extent.

White Bread

When whole wheat is refined to white flour, many vitamins and minerals are lost: vitamin B6 (72% loss), folic acid (67%), calcium (60%), magnesium (85%), manganese (86%), copper (68%), zinc (78%). Since grains make up about 30% of the average diet, consumption of refined grains depletes the total daily intake of micro-nutrients (vitamins and minerals).

Studies indicate that unfermented gluten consumption, whether from whole or refined grains, causes gut inflammation and subsequent mineral loss from bone.

Eat More Fruits and Vegetables

You are not vitamin deficient you are whole food deficient. Green leafy vegetables such as spinach and collard greens are especially good for maintaining healthy bones. Greater intake of fruits and vegetables is associated with a higher bone mineral density and a lower presence of osteoporosis.

Many fruits and vegetables contain a number of bone-friendly nutrients, including calcium, magnesium, potassium, vitamin K, vitamin C, and protein. Edible plants also provide anti-inflammatory agents and antioxidants, which counter inflammation and oxidative stress.

Eat Less Animal Protein

Planning a proper diet with balanced amount of every nutrient is one of the best natural ways to reverse osteoporosis. Excess intake of protein results in high level of acidity in the body, which further leads to calcium loss in the urine. It is better to refrain from consuming any protein in excess or more than the recommended amount to ensure the perfect musculoskeletal health.

Excessive dietary protein may promote bone loss. With

increasing protein intake, the urinary excretion of calcium also rises because calcium is mobilized to buffer the acidic breakdown products of protein. In addition, the amino acid methionine is converted to a substance called homocysteine, which is also apparently capable of causing bone loss.

Avoid Antacids

Stomach acid is vital in promoting absorption of minerals like zinc, magnesium and calcium in the body. However, indigestion, heartburn, reflux and peptic ulcer disease may compel people to take antacids. These drugs block the essential stomach acids, lessen mineral absorption in the body and thus increase the risk of osteoporosis. These drugs are meant to be consumed for only a very short period to limit the mineral loss. Restricting the use of antacids is one of the essential natural ways to reverse osteoporosis.

Get More Sunlight

Vitamin D is produced in the skin when the body gets exposed to sunlight. This essential vitamin is helpful in promoting efficient calcium absorption in the body and further putting this calcium in the bones. It also plays a vital role in strengthening and modulating the immune system of the body and fighting problems like depression and auto-immune disorders. However, skin cancer being a major cause of concern these days, people choose to apply sun screen on their body when they go out in the sun. Sun screen considerably limits the production of vitamin D in the body and consequently weakens the bones. In such cases, vitamin D supplements are essential to maintain required levels of the nutrient in the body.

Minerals

Required in numerous biochemical reactions in bone (connective) tissue minerals such as magnesium, manganese, boron, strontium, silicon, zinc, and copper. Silicon, for example, is found in high concentrations in growing bone. It strengthens connective tissue and may be crucial in osteoporosis prevention.

Minerals are found in rocks. The roots of plants pull the minerals into the plant making the minerals bio-available to us when we eat the plant food.

Calcium Supplements

While it is super important and the main component that makes up your bones, there is much misinformation when it comes to calcium too.

For starters, today we are told to intake higher than ever amounts of calcium, which almost all people find impossible to do unless they take a supplement.

Supplements, especially ones high in calcium or a form of calcium which is poorly digested, ends up creating more problems.

- For starters they throw off the body's natural calcium balance, which makes it harder for the body to absorb what it needs properly from food.
- Secondly, they lead to all sorts of problems in the kidneys, including kidney stones, as excess calcium is constantly trying to be filtered out.
- Thirdly, they increase problems with our cardiovascular health, and hardened calcium deposits can accumulate in the arteries.
- Fourthly, most calcium supplements cannot be absorbed into the bones and instead build up on the outside causing plaque and painful bone spurs.

So while I am not saying not to take a calcium supplement at all, I am also not saying to take one. There is much more research that needs to go in for each individual, whether they need a calcium supplement, what kind and how much. If you need a calcium supplement it is best to get a whole food calcium supplement which uses herbs and plant sources. Getting calcium from food sources is best as the body recognizes it and will use it or eliminate it if not needed.

Plant food rich in calcium include leafy greens, seeds, almonds, beans, lentils, legumes, dried fruit, and tofu. Sardines and canned salmon are loaded with calcium, thanks to their edible bones.

Magnesium

Magnesium is involved in over 300 metabolic reactions in the body. One of those involves bone metabolism. About 85% of the population is deficient in this mineral at the cellular level. Magnesium also balances calcium.

Magnesium is present in foods such as cocoa, seeds, nuts, and green leafy vegetables. Another good source of magnesium is Epsom salt. Prepare a hot water bath by pouring a cup of Epsom salt into the water and soak in the tub.

Eating magnesium-rich food and bathing in water stirred with Epsom salt are the best ways to acquire magnesium. But if your body fails to absorb magnesium in these two ways, then you can resort to supplements of magnesium to gain the benefits of magnesium.

So, make sure to include a good dose of magnesium into your diet. Eat foods rich in magnesium, consider taking supplements, and take baths in Epsom salt water to acquire the incredible health benefits of magnesium for bones. Don't forget to do your daily exercise because that is the essential thing that you do for your bone health.

Weight Bearing Exercise

Weight lifting, brisk walking using arm and leg weights, climbing stairs and hiking are some weight bearing exercises which can increase bone density effectively. Even 15 to 30 minutes of such exercises each day can do wonders for the body. Lifting weights, as small as 2 to 5 pounds, can also be extremely beneficial for the bones. Simple floor exercises like sit ups and leg lifts where one lifts their own body weight opposing gravity are very helpful too. Although exercises like cycling and swimming are very good for promoting fitness and muscle strength, these are not weight-bearing thus are not that beneficial for the bones. Planning properly structured weight lifting exercises is one of the most essential natural ways to reverse osteoporosis.

If you are sedentary the body doesn't bother to strengthen bones because it isn't necessary.

Build Up Bones With Walking

As you age, your bones become weaker. Luckily, you can strengthen your bones to ensure that they maintain their current condition if you walk more frequently. The low-impact exercise that you get when you walk will ensure that your bones retain their healthy density even as you age. If you retain your bone density, you'll significantly lower the odds of developing osteoporosis in your old age.

Fractures and other bone-related injuries will also decrease in frequency if you retain your bone density through regularly walking during both your youth and your golden years. Seeing as bones serve as the framework of the human body, healthier and stronger bones can increase stamina, improve balance, and give you good posture.

With each step you walk your feet continually pound on the ground and your body knows to build the bones stronger to accommodate the stress. If you are a couch potato your body does not build strong leg bones because they aren't being used, therefore there is no need.

Regularly walking can also decrease your chances of developing arthritis at any given point in your life. To summarize, your bones serve an important purpose in your body, many important purposes in fact, so it is your responsibility as the owner of your body to maintain its health by walking regularly.

Remember, getting older doesn't mean you have to suffer with brittle bones and debilitating diseases. These could be the best years of your life!

CHAPTER 12

Your Magical Immune System

"As you begin to heal the inner you, you alter your immune system." Wayne Dyer

Ignorance is the worst disease. We have been led to believe we need medical doctors and pharmaceutical medications to stay in good health. Nothing could be further from the truth, we have been incredibly misguided. Our power and knowledge of how our body works and heals has been taken from us. Big corporations profit from our lack of correct information.

We have been taught our health is preset by our genetics, and when we get older our bodies are going to break down and if cancer, diabetes, alzheimers, heart disease or obesity runs in our family there's nothing we can do about it. That's not true. It is a very disempowering belief that our health is predetermined by inherited genes. Your body is made to thrive, restore and regenerate itself and only succumbs to inherited problems when we don't properly care for them. Mostly what we inherit is an unhealthy lifestyle.

Science now says you can grow healthier and stronger with

each year that passes. You can grow new brain cells, build muscle and stronger bones. We just weren't taught how. We were taught a lie, that we have no control over our health, what we eat doesn't matter and we aren't qualified to take our health into your own hands.

When you treat your body right, over time it can grow a whole new healthier body by what you eat and how you live. In 10 years you have new bones, in 5 days the gut lining replaces itself and in 4 months you have new blood cells. If there is breath in your lungs and conscious thoughts in your mind it isn't too late to make changes to improve your health.

Western medicine has its place but daily health and preventative medicine is not their forte. Traditional doctors do their best to treat disease by relieving symptoms with pills, which may work for a short time, but pharmaceutical drugs taken over a long period of time weakens your immune system. Just like your muscles weaken when not used, your immune system weakens and gets lazy when pills take over its job. Drugs treat symptoms but they slowly kill your immune system making you sicker and stealing years from your life. Your immune system is the only thing that can heal you.

Where is the Immune System?

The immune system is spread throughout the body and involves many types of cells, organs, proteins, and tissues. The immune system is incredibly complicated and utterly vital for our survival. Several different systems and cell types work in perfect synchrony (most of the time) throughout the body to fight off pathogens and clear up dead cells.

Everyone's immune system is different but, as a general rule, it becomes stronger during adulthood as, by this time, we have been exposed to more pathogens and developed more immunity. That is why teens and adults tend to get sick less often than children.

Once an antibody has been produced, a copy remains in the body so that if the same antigen appears again, it can be dealt with more quickly.

Your immune system is dependent on the food you give it for nourishment. Healthy eating isn't confusing or complicated. The answer is always:

- Eat more plants and real whole foods; compounds in plants preform 1,000's of functions in the body.
- Eat less sugar, flour, processed food and meat.

You may think doctors would tell you food choices were important, if they really were. The truth is doctors learn next to nothing about nutrition in medical school. They can't teach you what they don't know. They are experts in disease management not health.

Food Choices for Immune Support

- Eat real food. Minimally processed, fresh fruits, vegetables, whole grains, legumes, nuts and seeds.
- Eat less. Mostly plants, which are nutrient dense and have more fiber than processed food.
- Eat mushrooms, they are anti-cancer
- Eat berries, fresh or frozen, they are loaded with phytonutrients and minerals.
- Eat beans, legumes, lentils and split peas. Soak them for 24 hours, drain and rinse, cover with fresh water and cook until soft.
- Eat greens and more greens. They are one food group in the world that will add years to your life.

- Use herbs and spices. Your spice cabinet is a medicinal pharmacy. Spices in different cultures have different health benefits.

Eat Less From a Box and More From the Earth

If you are new to eating this way don't let it intimidate you. Start with what you know you like. If you like cucumbers and green beans, great! Eat them everyday. Then make a commitment to try new fruits and vegetables and add in the ones you like to increase your intake.

The secret to a successful diet change is to slowly keep adding in more healthy choices, eventually crowding out the poor food choices. Slow works best for most people. Begin making small changes that are in alignment with your comfort level of commitment.

Tips:

- Explore new recipes. Find a few veggie-centric recipes that you love and keep them on a regular rotation.
- Soups are an excellent place to load up on veggies. Most start with a base of sauteed garlic and onion, it's easy to add extra veggies from there; think celery, carrots, potatoes, green beans, peppers, zucchini, kale, etc.
- Choose three or four of your favorite veggies to eat raw; carrots, cucumbers, bell peppers, radishes, cut them up and divide them into small storage containers that are easy to take on the go.
- Roast large batches of veggies to keep in the fridge for easy access throughout the week; beets, sweet potatoes,

broccoli, carrots, cauliflower. Warm or cold they are great added to salads, grain bowls or as a side dish.

- Toss in a handful of spinach or other greens into your smoothie, you'll never know they are there.
- There are many ways to eat a salad. Try adding diced up fruits, sprouts and nuts to your greens.
- Have a few vegetarian days per week, working you way up to a plant predominant diet.
- Plant based cooking is steaming, sauteeing, braising and roasting.
- Keep your fridge and freezer stocked with fruits and veggies so you'll always have quick options on hand.

This approach is easy to follow even for the person with no experience in the kitchen.

Mindful Eating

Mindful eating basically means that you take your time while eating and pay attention to what and how much of it you are putting in your body. In the wider sense, it means checking in with yourself before you eat to see if you're really hungry or are just having a craving or feeling a bit snacky. It also means learning to understand what your body needs and providing that, rather than having useless filler foods to silence your body's signals.

When you learn how to approach each day mindfully and listen to your body rather than the clock, calendar, and those around you, you are able to eat more sensibly.

I want to encourage you to look at your food a bit differently and take the time to really taste, enjoy and appreciate it. When you take a bite out of a juicy pear or have fresh, crisp lettuce, there are countless things going on in your body that many of us have stopped paying attention to. Feel the texture of that soft, juicy mango, the aroma of a fresh leaf of basil or cilantro, or the delicious flavor of a ripe red tomato. When you eat real food and enjoy the flavors and textures you will be less likely to make nutritionally poor food choices. By putting yourself in control of the food you eat, you will feel stronger and more empowered when it comes to your food choices.

Eating well is a form of self respect. Before you eat, take a moment to examine how you feel and express gratitude for your food. You wouldn't want to spend an hour cooking up a gorgeous dinner, only to have it disappear in 10 minutes, right? Whether you, a friend, or a five-star chef created the meal on your plate, take a moment to appreciate the love and ingredients that went into it. Savor the flavors, textures, and colors and treat it as you would your biggest indulgence. Plate your food in a beautiful way and it will be that much easier to savor and appreciate. When you're present and appreciative of what you are eating, you're more likely to be satisfied longer. When food is your friend, you can't help but feel happier.

Because it takes time for our stomachs to communicate how full it is with our brain, people who eat slowly tend to consume fewer calories than fast eaters. It is a good rule to chew a mouthful of food about 20 times before swallowing. Try to get in the habit of putting your fork down between bites. This may seem silly to do at every meal, but you'll find that over time, it will soon become the norm.

Digestion begins in the mouth, so the more work you do to chew before your food begins its journey, the more grateful your tummy will be later. Your stomach does not have teeth to do the work that needs to be done in the mouth.

No matter what, always check in with your fullness level. Stop when you are 80% full rather than eating until you can't eat anymore (100% or more). Your stomach is the size of your balled up fist. Keep that in mind when you look at your food portions.

Ensure you're keeping up your water intake throughout the

day as sometimes dehydration can be mistaken for hunger. You will usually eat less if you drink a glass of water 10 to 20 minutes before your meal.

Mindful Drinking

The beautiful, life affirming, healing properties of water can not be matched with anything else we put into our bodies. Look at every glass of water you drink as a way to add a healing intention into your body, infusing every single cell of every single tissue of every single organ system you have with healing support.

You can simply say a prayer, say an intention, even just think an intention as you hold your cup of water and silently bless it before you drink it.

However, if water is all you drink, you could be missing out on the health benefits of fresh fruits, vegetables and herbal teas. Don't get me wrong, drinking plenty of water is a good thing for everyone, however, it doesn't give you any antioxidants, phytonutrients, and other specific nutritional benefits.

Dehydration

Dehydration is life threatening. Severe dehydration means our organs absolutely can not function normally and leads to seizure, organ failure, and death. Dehydration can lead to or exacerbate common conditions such as constipation, dry skin, bad breath, headache, and high blood pressure.

- Humans, like Mother Earth, are made of 70% water. Every function of the body requires proper amounts of water. Every day our bodies turn over 2 - 2.5 liters (10 ½ cups) of water, losing most of this by respiration, perspiration, and excretion, and replacing the shortfall by the consumption of food and drink. But to truly thrive and live our best lives, some experts believe women really should be hydrating as much as 11 ½ cups (2.7 liters) a day.

- Having sluggish bowels is a classic symptom of chronic dehydration. Recent studies have shown that water status is the NUMBER ONE factor impacting regularity. More important than walking and more important that even fiber intake, water intake can turn constipation issues around completely.
- Dehydration causes the brain to shrink causing headaches, brain fog, forgetfulness and slow recall, brain and muscle tissues are water-rich. 83% of your lungs are water, the heart and the brain; 73% water, the bones; about 31% water, the kidneys and muscles; about 76% are water.
- Pain is actually a symptom of dehydration, often starting with a headache. I've literally had clients with a raging headache drink a glass of water and have the headache clear completely. The next time you have a headache or any type of pain, make sure you drink a glass of water and then re-evaluate your pain levels before reaching for a pain reliever or medication. Dehydration makes all pain worse, as the volume of the organs and joints deplete, dehydrated ligaments and cartilage get injured more easily and dehydrated discs in the spine allow increased pinching of nerves and muscle cramps increase as electrolytes deplete.
- Dehydration puts stress on the kidneys which inhibits filtration of our blood and cause infections.
- Dehydration also impacts your entire gut lining, and chronic dehydration can give rise to stomach ulcers and absorption issues as the mucosal layer stops secreting it's protective film.
- Not only does the gut lining need to be well hydrated to function, but also our entire respiratory lining does too. Our lungs absolutely require a moist mucous membrane to

function. In chronic dehydration, the mucus membranes in our respiratory system dry out and become more vulnerable to dust, pollen and other irritants. You may experience a dry cough as a result.

- Dehydration causes thick sticky blood which moves slowly through our veins and organs putting stress on our hearts to pump it through our body. If you have gone to a lab for a blood draw and they can't get your blood to flow into the tube they will send you off to drink water to thin your blood and when you return your blood is easily drawn. You were dehydrated and had thick sticky blood.
- When we decrease our water intake, our blood gets thicker making it harder to pump, our blood volume decreases, our heart rate increases and our blood vessels constrict. All together, this means your blood pressure raises and stays raised. If you are having blood pressure issues, it is more important than ever to be extremely vigilant about your hydration status.
- When our bodies are deprived of plain water, it causes blood to thicken and clot. Thick blood can't carry as much needed oxygen to the cells of the body. Drinking a glass before you go to bed and in the middle of the night offers more protection against heat attacks and strokes while you sleep, as it reduces the chances of becoming dehydrated.
- Plain water is readily absorbed, where other drinks have to first be filtered taking more energy and time to get water to cells that need it for optimal performance. Most medical doctor will give you a chemical blood thinner rather than advise you to drink more water and tell you how much you need to drink to keep your blood thin and flowing properly.
- How much water you need to drink daily depends on the weather, your activity level and how much fresh food and processed food you eat.

- The color and odor of your urine will tell you when you need more water. If you are adequately hydrated your urine will be very light yellow with no odor. The darker your urine gets and the stronger the odor gets, the more water you need to drink. As a general rule most people need one half of their body weight in ounces of water. Example: A 200-pound person will need 100 ounces of water daily.

Dehydration begins when we are just 1% volume depleted, but thirst doesn't set in until our body is about 2% volume depleted. By then we have already had effects on our mood, energy level, ability to think clearly, and pain levels. Instead of waiting for thirst or darkened urine to remind us to drink, let's utilize these preventative strategies for staying well hydrated, instead of treating dehydration.

What Makes Up The Immune System?

The immune system is confusing because it is a large system of defenses creating an internal environment through which our overall health is allowed to thrive and chronic diseases cannot.

Your immune system is made of up a complex collection of cells and organs. They all work together to protect you from germs and help you get better when you're sick. The main parts of the immune system are:

White blood cells: Serving as an army against harmful bacteria and viruses, white blood cells search for and attack and destroy germs to keep you healthy. White blood cells are the key part of the immune system. There are many white blood cell types in the immune system. Each cell type either circulates in the bloodstream and throughout the body or resides in a particular tissue, waiting to be called into action. Each cell type has a specific mission in your body's defense system. Each has a different way of recognizing a problem, communicating with other cells on the defense team and performing their function.

Lymph nodes: These small glands filter and destroy germs so they can't spread to other parts of your body and make you sick. They also are part of your body's lymphatic system. Lymph nodes contain immune cells that analyze the foreign invader brought to it and then activate, replicate and send the specific lymphocytes, which are white blood cells, to fight off that particular invader. You have hundreds of lymph nodes all over your body, including in your neck, armpits, and groin. Swollen, tender lymph nodes are a clue that your body is fighting an infection.

Spleen: Your spleen stores white blood cells that defend your body from foreign invaders. It also filters your blood, destroying old and damage red blood cells.

Tonsils and adenoids: Because they are located in your throat and nasal passage, tonsils and adenoids can trap foreign invaders (for example, bacteria or viruses) as soon as they enter your body. They have immune cells that produce antibodies that protect you from foreign invaders that cause throat and lung infections.

Thymus: This small organ in your upper chest beneath your breast bone helps mature a certain type of white blood cell. The specific task of this cell is to learn to recognize and remember an invader so that an attack can be quickly mounted the next time this invader is encountered.

Bone marrow: Stem cells in the spongy center of your bones develop into red blood cells, plasma cells and a variety of white blood cells and other types of immune cells. Your bone marrow makes billions of new blood cells every day and releases them into the bloodstream.

Skin, mucous membranes and other first-line defenses: Your skin is the first line of defense in preventing and destroying germs before they enter your body. Skin produces oils and secretes other protective immune system cells. Mucous membranes line the respiratory, digestive, urinary and reproductive tracts. These membranes secrete mucus, which lubricates and moistens surfaces. Germs stick to mucus in the respiratory tract and then are moved out of the airways by hair-like structures called cilia. Tiny hairs in your nose catch germs. Enzymes found in sweat, tears, saliva and mucus membranes as well as secretions in the vagina all defend and destroy germs.

Stomach and bowel: Stomach acid kills many bacteria soon after they enter the body. You also have beneficial (good) bacteria in your intestines that kill harmful bacteria. 80% of the immune system is in the intestines, referred to as the gut, colon and G.I. track (gastrointestinal). Your digestive system is a very good indicator of the health of your immune system.

Health is not just the absence of disease. It is an active state in our body protected by our own built-in defense systems so powerful they can actually reverse diseases like type 2 diabetes, heart disease and cancer. The immune system is an internal ecosystem that upholds life, rather than allowing it to collapse. Your immune system is the only thing that can heal you of physical ailments.

Boost Your Immune System With Vitamin C

Vitamin C has an immune-boosting effect that can help the body fight off illnesses, such as the common cold. One study found that vitamin C helped prevent pneumonia and supported tetanus treatment. Also, studies suggest that vitamin C plays a role in reducing lung inflammation that results from the flu.

Vitamin C is one of the most important vitamins your body requires and the only way to get Vitamin C is through diet. Almost all animals and plants synthesize their own Vitamin C but there are a few animals that cannot make their own vitamin C, including humans. Many of us are not eating enough Vitamin C-rich foods and our food supply contains less and less Vitamin C because of premature food harvesting, artificial ripening, and food processing.

Vitamin C has many important roles in the body, including supporting the production of collagen within the tissues. It also maintains the integrity of connective tissues; cartilage, capillaries, bones and teeth. When damage occurs to the body, Vitamin C helps rebuild the tissue and minimize scarring associated with the injury. It is involved in the biosynthesis of hormones.

Vitamin C also supports the immune system, it helps your body fight infections and reduces the effects of environmental pollutants. An extremely powerful antioxidant in itself, Vitamin C also helps regenerate other antioxidants like glutathione and vitamin E.

Vitamin C can help fight the effects of ageing, fight cancer and provide support for healing of all the body's cells. It may also be able to kill harmful bacteria, viruses, fungi and parasites within the body when present in sufficient concentrations. It helps fight the effects of flu, allergies and chemical exposure.

Known as the body's stress hormone, cortisol is produced in large amounts during stress to increase the mobilization of glucose from fats and proteins. It also stimulates appetite and is essentially the reason why some people prefer eating a lot of calories when they are stressed, a major risk factor for obesity. Some studies have shown that vitamin C can be helpful in reducing blood cortisol levels, including its synthesis from the adrenal glands. That's why vitamin C is so helpful in combating stress.

Pumping up your system with vitamin C is always a good idea.

Vitamin C Flush

A Vitamin C flush gives our system very, very high doses of vitamin C to the point where it totally saturates the system and in the process, brings the immune system up and supports rapid healing. This is ideal anytime you might be feeling run down, are recovering from illness or trauma/surgery, or your immune system simply needs a boost.

Recommended Ascorbic Acid For The Best Vitamin C Flush Results

For the most effective ascorbic acid flush, experts recommend that you take only a buffered vitamin C powder in the form of l-ascorbate. Buffered vitamin C powders contain a balancing blend of minerals including potassium, zinc, magnesium and calcium.

It's important to note that humans cannot absorb d-ascorbate, so be sure to get a powder that provides ascorbic acid in the form of l-ascorbate.

The reason you want a buffered vitamin C powder is because high doses of straight ascorbic acid can cause extreme acidity, irritation and/or inflammation of the lining in your gut.

Do the vitamin C flush on a day when you'll be home, comfortable and near a bathroom throughout the day.

To optimize the Vitamin C Flush, start in the morning on an empty stomach. Expect to cleanse for two to four hours, although for some people, more time is needed. Be sure to drink adequate water during the flush.

Take a spoonful in a half-glass of filtered/purified water or juice, every twenty to thirty minutes, keeping track of the total spoonfuls of ascorbic acid taken.

You may get a little bloated, or even a bit gassy towards the end, keep going until you actually pass a watery stool, this is the flush. Once you pass a very watery-stool, you can stop drinking the vitamin C solution.

After the Flush

Once the Vitamin C Flush is completed, you can continue taking smaller doses of ascorbic acid every four hours for the next couple days, trying to maintain a thicker, tapioca-like stool. If diarrhea occurs again, lower the dosage. This can be done for a more thorough detoxification, but is not required.

Once this level is reached your maintenance dose is 50% (or half) of the amount required for you to achieve a watery stool. Your maintenance dose should be maintained until you are feeling better, your symptoms have improved, your stress has reduced, or whatever was causing the low vitamin C has been improved.

A Vitamin C Flush can be done as often as once a month or once every four months.

The healthier your body is, the less vitamin C you will require, the more vitamin C it takes to flush your system the more your body NEEDS vitamin C. Always remember to stay hydrated during this process by drinking plenty of water.

Foods High in Vitamin C

When most people think about vitamin C, the image of an orange suddenly appears in their mind. However, it is not only citrus fruits that contain vitamin C, and many different foods are good sources of it.

Some fruits that are good sources of vitamin C include:

- Guava
- Citrus Fruits
- Kiwi

- Strawberries
- Blueberries
- Aamla or Indian Gooseberry
- Tomatoes
- Cantaloupe/melons

Some vegetables that are good sources of vitamin C include:

- Red and green bell pepper
- Broccoli
- Brussels sprouts
- Tomato juice
- Cabbage
- Sweet potato
- Cauliflower
- Collards
- Turnip greens
- Kale
- Chili peppers
- Leafy greens
- Potatoes
- Raw herbs like cilantro, basil, mint, tarragon, chives, dill

To get the most vitamin C, eat a variety of raw fruits and vegetables every day. Vitamin C is necessary for good health. Because it is abundant in many plant foods, eating a healthful diet that includes a variety of fruits and vegetables usually provides a person with all the vitamin C that they need. All you have to do is eat real food.

Get A Handle On Your Stress

Because chronic stress can weaken your immune system, here are suggestions to bring down your stress levels:

- Do daily relaxation techniques such as yoga, meditation and mindfulness breathing exercises. You can find guided applications on YouTube.
- Take a warm bath or shower in the evening; savor a cup of herbal tea.
- Exercise when you can. Exercise boosts your immune system by flushing bacteria out of your lungs and airways, helping your antibodies and white blood cells fight disease.
- Go on a daily walk for 20-30 minutes.
- Like diet and exercise, quality sleep has a profound impact on our physical, emotional and mental well-being. Don't try to stay up late to catch up on work. Give yourself a firm lights-out time. Try to go to bed and wake up around the same time every day, including weekends. This helps establish your sleep/wake cycle (a.k.a. your circadian rhythm).
- Prioritize your to-do list into "Has to be done now" and "Can wait."
- Learn to say no to added responsibilities. You can only do so much.
- Stay in touch with the positive people in your life, the ones you know who will support you, listen to you and make you laugh.

CHAPTER 13

Blood Sugar and Type II Diabetes

Sugar is now more dangerous than gunpowder

A diet which is high in calorie, fat and sugar content when eaten long term can lead to obesity and its complications, namely, atherosclerosis, hypertension, heart disease and diabetes. These conditions predispose an individual to insulin resistance, where the fat, muscle and other cells cannot absorb and utilize glucose from the blood for energy.

A sedentary lifestyle added to an unhealthy diet increases your risk of type2 diabetes. As sitting time is increased, so is the risk for type 2 diabetes and other chronic diseases; what's more, even if you exercise regularly for 30 minutes a day you are still at a higher risk for diabetes if you sit for more than four hours a day. Sitting for more than six hours a day increases the risk for cancer, heart disease, and high blood pressure.

Every two hours you spend sitting in front of the television increases your risk for type 2 diabetes by 14 percent, according to the Harvard School of Public Health. You don't need to exercise every half-hour, but you should stand up, stretch, and move around for a few minutes.

Diabetes prevention is possible as long as you make changes to eliminate risk factors. You can get started by doing the following:

- Eat a healthy diet.
- Get to a healthy weight and stay there.
- Start a regular exercise program and stick with it. Walking briskly for 30 minutes every day cuts your diabetes risk by 30 percent.
- Cut back on your sitting time, turn off that TV and get up and get moving!
- Don't smoke.
- Drink alcohol only in moderation. That means no more than one drink a day.

Type 2 diabetes is caused by years of a poor diet and inactivity and can be reversed with a healthy diet, movement and healthy lifestyle choices.

Healing Type 2 Diabetes With a Raw Food Diet

You have probably heard that diabetes has no cure, just the possibilities of a variety of complications. This is an old belief system backed by many medical professionals and pharmaceuticals who band-aid this disease.

Since the 1920's, live-food nutrition has been used to heal diabetes naturally since Dr. Max Gerson healed Dr. Albert Schweitzer of his Type-2 diabetes using this diet. Plant-based live-food nutrition worked then, and it still works today.

Fresh fruits and vegetables are the mainstays of the plan, and are accompanied by nuts, seeds, seaweed, grains, legumes, nut milks and water. Omitting preparation methods that involve cooking leave the acceptable items prepared by methods like dehydrating, blending, juicing, soaking and sprouting. Although preparation methods vary, many of the foods recommended on a raw food diet for diabetes are healthy, whole foods.

Proponents of the cooking-free plan argue that it's the best diabetic diet for several reasons.

- Obviously, there are substantial weight loss benefits to be gained from only eating whole, fresh foods and nothing else. Weight loss can be a huge factor in helping to better manage diabetes.
- Additionally, nutritional benefit from eating uncooked foods can be substantial, with often forgotten about vitamins and minerals being available in great quantity when consumed in the foods that contain them.
- Raw vegetables carry fiber content that helps the body absorb sugar more slowly.
- Green leafy vegetables like spinach contain natural chemicals that might help reduce blood sugar levels.
- Many fresh fruits that are a staple of a raw food diet for diabetes, such as blueberries, boast natural compounds that are thought to help reduce blood sugar levels high above where they should be when enjoyed as a part of a sensible meal or snack.
- Digestive benefits, improvement to the feel and appearance of skin and hair, and prevention of disease like heart problems and cancer are all also thought to be potential benefits of a raw food diet for diabetes.

Therefore, not only might a raw food diet for diabetes promote weight loss, it's also an opportunity to gain important natural benefits.

This disease reversal demands that dedication to diet and

exercise be maintained in order to prevent a resurgence in the disease, but proves how powerful diet and physical activity can be. A raw food diet for diabetes might just be the ideal solution because it promotes energy which leads to more physical activity, supports healthy weight loss and contains the nutritional content the body needs to properly manage its blood sugar levels.

Factor this information into your personal Divine Diet if you are predisposed to atherosclerosis, hypertension, heart disease and diabetes. Get your Goddess body back on track.

Can't Kick the Sugar?

Sugary and fatty foods affect the pathways to the brain in the same way as heroin or cocaine. Sugar acts directly in the brain to inhibit the effect of leptin and increased appetite so you never feel full. So then you keep eating, and you become leptin-resistant. What you need to do is break the addiction by detoxing the liver, which has stopped metabolizing fat properly.

Sugar consumption causes fat to build up in liver cells, which decreases the liver's ability to metabolize fats and sugars and detoxify your body.

You can take some supplements to help with sugar withdrawal and carb cravings: Chromium picolinate, 1,000 mg daily can help with sugar withdrawal. Vitamin B complex, 100 percent daily allowance, helps with carbohydrate cravings.

The Body Will Heal and Repair Itself

There are many ways to accomplish the same end, there is no ONE way for everyone. Find your way and believe in with all your heart and your body will too.

I am using diabetes as just one example of how the body will heal and repair itself if you give it what it needs; a plant predominant diet and take away what is harming it; a processed toxic diet.

Before turning to prescription drugs and other man-made treatments, numerous common medical conditions and diseases can be cured or healed through nature. A variety of herbs, minerals, vitamins, lifestyle changes, and exercise can help the body and mind achieve a renewed sense of health.

Disease, dis-ease, can manifest in many ways. Getting to the root of the problem will always be the same, with a few variances:

- A plant predominant diet
- Hydration with clean water
- Physical activity
- A healthy digestive system
- Sunshine, fresh air, walking on the earth
- Rest
- An organic mindset
- Nutritional supplements for particular issues
- Extreme self-care

CHAPTER 14

Healthy Digestive System

Digestion is one of the most delicately balanced of all human and perhaps angelic functions.

Death begins in the colon and an unhealthy colon is the root cause behind many health problems. This was believed to be the case by Hippocrates, a famous ancient Greek physician (ca. 460 BC – ca. 370 BC). Modern science has shown that he was correct. More than 50 million Americans have bowel issues related to colon health. While some of the problems are relatively minor, many others are very serious illnesses. They include:

- Acid Reflux
- Bloating / Gas
- Heartburn / Indigestion
- Constipation / Diarrhea
- Mood Swings
- Depression / Fatigue
- Foggy Brain
- Headaches
- Skin Problems

- Food Intolerance
- Colitis
- Crohn's Disease
- Irritable Bowel Syndrome
- Leaky Gut
- Auto Immune Disease
- Rheumatoid Arthritis

Besides these serious colon problems, colon issues lead to colostomy surgery for more than 100,000 people each year. Some healthcare professionals say the average person has between 5 and 20 pounds of waste matter stuck in their colon for nearly 70 hours when healthy digestive systems should process food in under 24 hours. As a result, up to 80% of disease and abdominal discomfort people suffer may be related to toxic colons. Part of the problem is that the processed fast food diets many people eat today lack natural fibers and enzymes, and have too much fat and refined sugar.

Have you noticed that modern convenience has abandoned traditional foods? Most of what is available to eat today, whether from the market or restaurant, is either highly processed or made with ingredients that are themselves highly processed. What do we lose when we stop eating traditional foods? In a word, our health! Our health begins in the gut.

Weight Gain

When digestion is unhealthy and the stomach and intestines are overloaded with toxicity from the standard modern diet and environmental exposures, the human body pads the vital organs with extra visceral and subcutaneous fat as a protective defense. In other words, the waistline grows. It may be that a healthier digestive system negates the need for the body to start padding organs with extra fat.

Gut Health Affects Mental Health

Taking care of our mental and emotional issues is more controllable than you think. Poor health keeps you in a very dense, low vibrating energy of fear, anxiety and depression.

For those suffering from psychological symptoms, it can seem like a losing battle. Don't throw up your hands just yet, the factors with the most determination in your mental health are more controllable than you think. If you already suffer from digestive issues, it's imperative that you heal your gut and get your body back in balance in order to maintain your psychological health.

The key to treating many of the most common psychological symptoms is recognizing that most are actually rooted in your gut, not your brain. The goal should be to restore the balance of your intestinal flora by treating infections, inflammation, parasites, candida and avoiding problematic foods.

The best antidepressant is a healthy whole food diet and a high potency probiotic to fuel a healthy gut microbiome. Keep in mind a probiotic pill cannot take the place of a healthy diet, it is a supplement and assists a good diet.

Certainly there are some psychological conditions that do not originate from gut imbalances alone. Post Traumatic Stress Disorder, Bipolar Disorder, and other major conditions have significant genetic and environmental components.

Medication and certain therapies might be necessary in addition to fixing the gut in order to maintain a high quality of life. However, the vast majority of psychological complaints suffered by the general population such as brain fog, anxiety, depression, mood swings, and concentration issues are rooted in neurotransmitter imbalances that begin in the gut.

So how do these imbalances occur? Most people can attribute their symptoms to one or all of these causes: infections, too many rounds of antibiotics and food sensitivities.

Conventional western medicine views the body in distinct systems and psychological stressors as independent from the rest of the body, but in actuality our brains are inextricably tied to our gastrointestinal tract. This is because 90-95% of our serotonin, a key neurotransmitter responsible for regulating mood, is made in our gut. A deficiency in serotonin causes depression and in some, anxiety, in fact, the majority of antidepressants work by blocking the brain's serotonin receptors, freeing up more of the chemical to remain present in the brain. Serotonin and other vital neurotransmitters travel from the gut to the brain via the vagus nerve, the longest nerve that emerges directly from the brain.

Because chemical signals travel both from the gut to the brain and vice versa, those with gastrointestinal symptoms are at a higher risk of mood imbalances, anxiety, and depression. In order to solve the problem, or prevent future symptoms, you must address the root cause: something is happening in the gut to suppress your ability to make your serotonin.

How to Heal the Gut

"All disease starts in the gut" Hippocrates

As with all health concerns, there is no one-size-fits-all approach for healing the gut. It is a complex web that needs to be approached from a holistic and functional perspective. But without addressing diet and lifestyle factors, you will not be able to recover. So start today by taking baby steps, or jumping in whole hog, whichever method works best for you. Respect your digestive tract and you will set the stage for whole-body wellness.

Since the gut houses so much of your immune system &

immune response, it's an important place to look when you're dealing with chronic illness and inflammation. We are increasingly bombarded with substances such as pesticides, heavy metals, etc. that damage the sensitive, porous lining of the gut.

Drink a Ton of Water

The first and most important remedy is water and a lot of it. If it is the only thing you do, increase your water consumption. Water will hydrate, lubricate, moisten and flush out all 30 feet of your intestines. It will aid in removing blockages and nests of parasites hiding in old fecal matter. It will allow your intestinal lining to self repair and absorb the nutrients into your blood stream.

Adding fresh lemon to your water will improve the taste, add needed minerals to your water, help alkalize your fluids and aid your liver.

Spa Water Recipes

Jazz up your daily hydration with infused flavored water. Add loads of flavor and healthy nutrients by adding fresh fruits and herbs to your pitcher. Unlike commercially bottled products, homemade vitamin water contains no added sugar, no artificial sweeteners, and no added weirdness. And seeing a beautiful jar of deliciousness sitting in the fridge is like a work of art!

Fill up a half-gallon Mason jar or pitcher with water flavorings, ice and water in the morning, with a goal of getting through it twice in a day. That's roughly 120 ounces of water, or 15 glasses a day. The flavoring fruits, veggies and herbs will easily get you through two jar fill-ups and still keep their flavor. And in fact, I usually use them for two or more days. Basically, when they lose their flavor, I toss them in the compost and start over with a new combo. But until then, I just keep on filling it up!

Cucumbers, Lime, Strawberries and Fresh Mint

In a half-gallon jar, or a 2 quart pitcher, layer the strawberries, cucumbers, lime slices, and mint leaves. Add ice cubes. Fill jar or pitcher with water. Let chill for 10 minutes, and then enjoy!

Obviously, the longer the water sits, the stronger the flavor. It's mild at first, but after a few hours (or overnight) it's quite strong.

- Soft fruits like strawberries and peaches need to be sliced to release their flavors.
- Herbs need to be fresh, they can be crushed a bit to release their essential oils and aromas.
- Citrus can be peeled or not, but steeped too long they can get bitter.
- Fresh or frozen fruit can be used.

More Spa Water Combinations:

- lemons and blueberries
- blackberries and sage
- lemon and mint
- cucumber and lemon and basil
- grapefruit and rosemary
- pineapple and mint
- watermelon and rosemary
- cinnamon and pear and ginger
- strawberries and lavender
- nectarine and basil and clementines
- rosemary and ginger
- grapefruit and coriander
- sliced apple and cinnamon sticks
- tangerine and thyme
- peach and ginger
- sliced grapes and mint

- sliced blood orange, 5 whole cloves and 2 whole star anise
- citrus and cucumber
- pear and fennel
- strawberries and lemon and grapefruit

Chew Your Food!

Although there is some debate when it comes to digestion, overall you will get more nutrients and greater health benefits from food in its most natural, raw state. There have been claims that raw food causes digestive issues and bloating. If this is an issue for you try increasing the number of times that you chew your food before swallowing. The optimal amount of "chews" have been listed between 50 to 80 depending on the food you're eating. Think about it like this,the more digestion done in your mouth, the easier it will be for the digestion in your stomach!

Proper digestion starts in your mouth. When eating, be sure to chew your food thoroughly to get the full benefit out of it. By focusing on chewing many times, you will eat slower. This can improve your digestion, help you eat less, and enhance your overall eating experience.

Saliva is extremely important for your health. As soon as you eat and chew your food, extra saliva is produced. This saliva allows your food to fall apart into tiny pieces. There is a substance, an enzyme in your saliva called amylase. Amylase helps with the digestion of starch in bread and potatoes, for example. Your body can normally not digest starch well, but when it is mixed with saliva, amylase begins the process and you have less trouble with this later on in your stomach and intestines.

When you chew well, the food turns into smaller pieces and the amylase is more effective. Later, in your stomach and intestines, more food is digested and processed, giving you a stronger feeling of satisfaction. You feel less like eating something else. Compare it to a handful of nuts. If you don't chew the nuts well, you poop most of them out. If you chew the nuts until they are fine, your body can extract more nutrition from them and you feel fuller.

The goal is to chew the food until its texture is similar to that of a well-blended smoothie, whether that takes 20 chews, 32 chews or 40 chews or more for raw food. There isn't a magic number, just the right texture. Foods that are harder to chew, such as steak and nuts, may require up to 40 chews per mouthful. Foods like watermelon may require fewer chews to break down, as few as 10 to 15.

When large particles of food don't break down all the way in your stomach, because you didn't take the time to chew them, they can continue on into your intestines. When this occurs, the food can start to putrefy, which can cause excess bacteria in the gut and an overall less healthy gut environment.

You don't have teeth in your stomach! Chew your food in your mouth before it hits your stomach and causes digestive stress through your whole system.

Chewing is the first step of digestion:

- Chewing and saliva break down and mix food together in your mouth. From there, food goes into your esophagus when you swallow.
- Your esophagus pushes food into your stomach.
- Your stomach holds food while it mixes with enzymes that continue breaking down the food so you can use it for energy.
- When food is digested enough in your stomach, it moves into your small intestine where it mixes with more enzymes that continue to break it down. Nutrients from the food are absorbed in the small intestine.
- Wastes are sent to the large intestine, known as your colon. The leftover waste is excreted through the rectum and anus.

Here are some tips for how to eat to improve your digestive health:

- Drink 30 minutes before or after you eat, but not with your meal. This increases the efficiency of your digestion.
- Don't drink coffee right after a meal. That can speed up your digestion and send you to the bathroom. It can also cause heartburn from its acidity.
- Avoid fruits and processed sweets right after a meal. Sugary foods are digested quickly and may cause gas and bloating.
- Avoid exercising strenuously after a meal. Digestion requires energy, and it's less efficient when you're exercising.
- Eat more fermented foods like sauerkraut and pickles. They contain digestive enzymes and beneficial bacteria needed to help your body absorb essential nutrients.
- Eat raw or slightly steamed vegetables, which contain higher amounts of enzymes and fiber. These are important for good digestion.
- Go for a walk after a meal. This speeds the rate at which food moves through your intestines, aiding digestion.

Portion Size

Portion size is just as important as the food itself. Your stomach is the size of your balled-up fist. Look at the food on your plate and imagine how much of it would fit into your closed fist, if it were chewed up, and limit your portion to that much. It will take a few weeks but your stomach will shrink and you won't want to eat large portions anymore.

American portion sizes are too big, so are most Americans. We are gluttons and don't even know it. An example is; your meat and fish serving should be the size of a deck of cards, not take up half of the plate.

Typically, we aren't operating at a high vibrational frequency when we're too full. Instead, we're pushing negative feelings or emotions away and numbing out with food which lowers our vibrational frequency to not feel anything. Be Divine, eat less.

Regular Bowel Movements

If constipation is an issue, there are supplements to consider for a temporary fix:

- Magnesium Citrate: Magnesium is a mineral that is critical for energy production and metabolism. It encourages muscle contraction, which often causes bowel movements regularly.
- Psyllium Husk Powder: Husk Powder is a fine-textured organic product high in natural fiber made for mixing in your food or beverages. It is very absorbent and promotes regularity and overall digestive health.
- Smooth Move Tea: This herbal tea, and others, relieves occasional constipation with the combination of Senna, a laxative herb and peppermint for extra digestive support. Best taken at bedtime for regular mornings. This same formula is also available as a capsule if you want the benefits of herbal tea without the slightly bitter taste of Senna.

Add more fibrous whole food to your diet to accelerate elimination. When toxic waste is slow moving and stuck in your body it not only causes stress, acidity and disease but ages you considerably.

Your food should be broken down, nutrients absorbed and waste eliminated, within 24 hours. What you ate yesterday should eliminated today. When you eat a meal it should push through to help you eliminate a previous meal, which is why it is normal to feel you need to have a bowel movement after you eat.

You can determine the health of your digestive system by your bowel movements:

- If you ate 3 meals yesterday, you should have 3 bowel movements today.
- Your poo should not stink, it will have a slight odor but not be rank. The worse the odor, the slower the transit time and your food is rotting and purifying inside your body.
- Your elimination should be brown, not white or yellow or black.
- Shaped like a log, not runny (your body doesn't like what you ate) or like rabbit pellets (you are dehydrated)
- Easily eliminated, not strained (you need more water and fiber)
- Float on the water, if it sinks you need more fiber, if it floats you ate enough fiber yesterday. Congratulations! Do it again! I get phone calls with the first words out of my clients mouth is "It floated!" It takes diligence to heal your digestive system and it is something to be proud of.

Bottom Line (yes that's a pun)

- 2 to 3 bowel movements per day
- Easy elimination
- Very little odor
- Shaped like a log
- Brown in color
- Floating on the water

Make it a habit to look at your bowel movements and pay attention to what they are telling you.

When your doctor tells you it is normal to only have a bowel movement every few days, it is a lie! If you are taking medication that causes constipation you have to be more diligent working with your food, fiber, exercise, water consumption and possibly supplements to get things moving. It is not ok to be backed up reabsorbing toxins that need to be eliminated. Take a good look at your B.M.'s and see what you are eliminating which you were carrying around inside of you! You want to get rid of that A.S.A.P.

Intestinal Flora

Also called gut flora, microbiota, microflora and microbiome, these organisms consist of bacteria, fungi, protozoa and yeast, and have specific purposes that help the body. Not only do intestinal flora work to help the body break down and digest foods, they also are responsible for synthesizing some types of vitamins and nutrients. For example, normal intestinal flora help the body create vitamin K. They also provide assistance with mineral absorption and work to change some types of starches and sugars into sources of energy for the body.

Healthier Gut Bacteria

The good bacteria that make up your intestinal flora live and flourish off fiber. As your gut bacteria gobble up fiber that has fermented in your G.I. tract, they produce short-chain fatty acids that have a host of benefits-including lowering systemic inflammation, which has been linked to obesity and nearly every major chronic health problem. A recent Italian study found that eating a high-fiber Mediterranean diet was associated with higher levels of short-chain fatty acids. "And you can start to see the changes in gut bacteria within just a few days," says Kelly Swanson, Ph.D., a professor of nutritional sciences at the

University of Illinois at Urbana-Champaign. The catch: You've got to consistently get enough grams, ideally every day, if not most days of the week, to keep getting the benefits. Skimping on fiber shifts bacteria populations in a way that increases inflammation in the body.

Considering that our daily diet is made up of a patchwork of foods that pass our lips, just pause for thought next time you eat something, and consider whether it's going to purposefully contribute to your daily 30 grams of fiber goal.

Thankfully, there are so many delicious high-fiber foods out there that will help you hit your fiber goal in no time. While apples may be our first thought when thinking of high-fiber foods to add to your diet, a medium-sized apple has 4 grams, there are plenty of other options that will give you even more fiber bang for your buck.

The good bacteria need fiber, fermented and whole foods to flourish and outnumber the bad bacteria which thrives on sugar and flour. Eating a poor diet of refined, processed food upsets the balance of intestinal flora negatively affecting the health of your whole body, to include your weight, immune system and brain health.

Indigenous people have had many different diets throughout history, depending on their environment. What they had in common was that they ate large amounts of fiber.

Foods High in Fiber

Berries: While all berries are a healthy choice, raspberries (and blackberries) come out on top with just under 9 grams of fiber per cup, not to mention a healthy dose of vitamin C. While still delicious and fiber-rich, strawberries have only 3 grams of fiber per cup and blueberries have 4 grams.

Black Beans: A 1/2-cup serving of black beans offers a hefty 8 grams. That's nearly one-third of the daily fiber recommendation for women. Black beans are also a great source of protein, with 7 grams per serving. Rinse canned beans prior to use to help reduce the sodium.

Avocados: Beyond their heart-healthy fats and super-delicious taste, there is even more reason to love avocados-there are about 7 grams of fiber in half an avocado.

Artichokes: When you think of fiber, artichokes might not be one of the first foods that come to mind, but they should be. 1 cup of cooked artichoke hearts contains 6 grams of fiber! Artichokes are also a good source of potassium, a mineral and electrolyte which is important for heart function and can help maintain normal blood pressure.

Lentils: A member of the legume family, lentils are extremely versatile and have a tender bite when cooked. And, 1/2 cup of cooked lentils delivers around 8 grams of fiber.

Sweet Potatoes: This favorite fall tuber offers 5 grams of fiber in a medium spud. Sweet potatoes also deliver vitamin A, an important vitamin for healthy vision and immune function.

Chickpeas: This little legume delivers a big fiber punch. There are about 6 grams of fiber in 1/2 cup of cooked chickpeas. Also called garbanzo beans, chickpeas are a vegan-friendly source of protein.

Oatmeal: For a fiber-rich and filling breakfast, reach for oatmeal. A 1/2 cup of cooked oats has just under 5 grams of fiber and is a satisfying whole grain.

Green Peas: Peas are finally starting to get the recognition they deserve for being a plant-protein powerhouse, but they are also a great source of fiber. A standard 2/3 cup serving of green peas offers 6 grams, making them the perfect ingredient to sneak in your family's favorite dinner dishes.

Fiber Magic

Fiber has such a huge impact on gut health, which in turn has profound effects on both physical and mental health. Within our gut, we have around 4 1/2 pounds of microbes that digest our food and regulate our nervous system, our immune system, and other vital organs. Poor nutrition such as daily intake of high sugar foods or processed foods can wreak havoc with these microbes in our gut, increasing the likelihood of metabolic diseases such as obesity, Type 2 diabetes, and heart disease.

Increase Fiber: As adults we should consume 30 grams of fiber per day, that is 2 tablespoons or 1/4 cup, yet most of us only achieve 18 grams. More than 95 percent of Americans don't consume enough fiber on a daily basis, and that's a serious problem for so many aspects of our health. Women should aim for at least 25 grams of fiber each day, while men should shoot for at least 38 grams.

However, the easiest way to know if you have eaten enough fiber, to do all of the things fiber needs to do, is to look at your bowel movements. If your stool floats today, you ate enough fiber yesterday. If it sinks like a submarine, you did not eat enough fiber yesterday and you need to immediately increase it.

Fiber can only be found naturally in whole, plant-based foods like whole grains, fruits, veggies, nuts, seeds and legumes.

Want to increase the fiber in your diet? Start by making realistic, small tweaks:

- Swap out your refined grains for whole varieties
- Serve a side salad with dinner
- Add a handful of berries or an apple to your breakfast each morning
- Add chia seeds to yogurt or juices
- Add flax seeds to smoothies
- Make overnight oatmeal cups for breakfast

Little changes like that can make a huge difference.

Just make sure you're drinking plenty of fluids to help all this additional fiber pass through the body! As fiber passes through the stomach and intestines, it absorbs water, adding bulk to the stool. This promotes regularity and reduces constipation. Fiber naturally scrubs and promotes the elimination of toxins from your G.I. tract.

Too much fiber can cause diarrhea, not enough can cause constipation and just the right amount will cause your bowel movements to float, if they sink you need more fiber.

Insoluble Fiber: Insoluble fiber, found in wheat bran, whole grains, fruits and vegetables, speeds the passage of food through the stomach and intestines. Because insoluble fiber makes things move along more quickly, it limits the amount of time that chemicals like BPA, mercury and pesticides stay in your system. The faster they go through you, the less chance they have to cause harm.

Soluble Fiber: Soluble fiber found in oat bran, barley, oranges, apples, carrots, and dried beans, turns into a gel during the digestive process and prevents cholesterol, fat, and sugars from being absorbed by the body. Soluble fiber soaks up potentially harmful compounds, such as excess estrogen and unhealthy fats, before they can be absorbed by the body.

Pectin

One of the most powerful foods on the planet for healing leaky gut and reversing antibiotic damage is none other than stewed apples. This source of pectin is an easily accessible fuel that your gut cells can instantly use to heal and regenerate. Apple pectin has the ability to sweep out radioactive dust particles from the intestinal tract, and it was used extensively after the Chernobyl nuclear plant meltdown.

Taking a Probiotic Supplement

If you're NOT eating a balanced, whole-food diet, supplementing with probiotics won't do a lot of good. An isolated supplement can't fix a broken diet. Address your diet first, then add probiotics to aid in healthier gut flora, especially after taking a round of antibiotics.

Antibiotics

Antibiotics from a prescribed pill kill off the good gut bacteria as well as the bad bacteria. The stronger antibiotics we need the more good bacteria it kills, the immune system is weakened and sicker we become. After the round of medication is finished, you need to reseed your gut with new, good bacteria in a probiotic supplement.

We also get a steady stream of antibiotics from commercially prepared meat like chicken, beef or pork and dairy products causing our bodies to build up an immunity to them, which creates super bugs that become resistant to antibiotics when we may really need it. One more reason to eat only organic, no hormones, no antibiotic, no GMO meat or factory farmed dairy products.

Mono Meals

A mono meal is a meal which is composed of only one type of fruit or vegetable. This means that you eat only watermelon for a meal and nothing else. Or just cherries and nothing else. Or bananas and nothing else. The most wonderful thing about eating fruit is the simplicity of it, it is nature's original fast food. Imagine a beautiful, juicy nectarine or sweet strawberry, juicy mango. Just take it, wash it and bite it and you will taste the explosion of flavors, which is in a mature, high-quality fruit.

None of the animals in the wild cook food and no animal prepares their meals with several ingredients, such as we do. A really good fruit really cannot be improved, because it is already perfect. Mother Nature has done that.

Things are greatly simplified if you consume only one type of food at a time, because you only need to create digestive juices for only this type of food and your digestion can fully concentrate on it. A mono meal is the easiest meal on your digestive system.

When you eat only one type of food at a time, you give special emphasis to chewing, taste and texture, that is why your body will clearly let you know when it is no longer hungry and when it is time to stop eating. Delicious food that you were eating a moment ago will suddenly be tasteless and unappealing, making it almost impossible to overeat.

When your taste buds become accustomed to simple mono meals, you will no longer need various toppings, spices or heat treatment in order to enjoy it. You will learn to appreciate food in its most natural state.

Healing Broths

Broth is rich in minerals to strengthen the immune system and support healthy digestion. Bone broths have been the rage for the last few years and all the "experts" have jumped on the band wagon, but there isn't anything in bone broth you can't also get in vegetable and herb broths.

The most beneficial nutrients and electrolytes in bone broth can be found in vegan-friendly sources and the one thing that sets itself apart, the thing that is impossible for vegans to find a veggie replacement for is the collagen. However, plants offer richer sources in collagen building blocks and, in addition, provide nutrients not found in sufficient quantities in meats or broth. There are many other foods that have been shown to contribute towards healing the stomach lining and digestive tract, such as seaweed, aloe vera, healthy fats and turmeric.

Broth "Gut Healing" Recipes

Mineral Broth

Makes 6 quarts

Ingredients:

- 1 fennel bulb, plus tops
- 2 unpeeled yellow onions, cut into quarters
- 6 unpeeled carrots, cut into thirds
- 1 leek, white and green parts, cut into thirds
- 1 bunch celery, including the heart, cut into thirds
- 2 unpeeled sweet potatoes, washed and cut into chunks
- 1 garnet yam, washed and cut into chunks
- 1 large bunch fresh, flat-leaf parsley
- 6 sprigs fresh thyme
- 12 large cloves unpeeled garlic, cloves smashed
- 3 inches unpeeled ginger, cut in half, lengthwise
- 1/8 inch strip of kombu
- 12 black peppercorns
- 4 juniper berries or allspice berries

- 2 bay leaves
- 8 quarts cold, filtered water
- 1 teaspoon sea salt

Directions:

Rinse all the vegetables well, including the kombu. In a 12-quart or larger stock pot, combine the onions, carrots, leek, celery, sweet potatoes, parsley, thyme, garlic, ginger, kombu, peppercorns, juniper berries, and bay leaves. Fill the pot with 8 quarts of water, cover and bring to a boil.

Remove the lid, decrease the heat to low and simmer, uncovered, for 2 to 4 hours. As the broth simmers, some of the water will evaporate; add more if the vegetables begin to peek out. Simmer until the full richness of the vegetables can be tasted.

Strain the broth through a large, course-mesh sieve (remember to use a heat-resistant container underneath), then add salt to taste. Let cool to room temperature before refrigerating or freezing.

Variation: For an extra immune boost, add 8 shitake mushrooms to the stock and/or a six inch piece of Burdock root, washed and cut into quarters.

Notes:
Store refrigerated in an airtight container for 5 to 7 days or in the freezer for 4 months.

Balancing the broth: A squeeze of lemon juice and some sea salt, about 1/8 teaspoon of each per cup, does a lot to bring this broth to life.

Like fine wine, this broth gets better with age. A longer simmer will increase the broth's taste and nutrient density. You can also cut the recipe in half and make it in a slow cooker.

Gut Healing Vegetable Broth

Ingredients:

- 12 cups / 2 3/4 litres filtered water
- 1 tbsp coconut oil, or extra-virgin olive oil, optional
- 1 red onion, quartered (with skins)
- 1 garlic bulb, smashed
- 1 chilli pepper, roughly chopped (with seeds)
- 1 thumb-sized piece of ginger, roughly chopped (with skin)
- 1 cup greens, such as kale or spinach
- 3-4 cup mixed chopped vegetables and peelings, I used carrot peelings, red cabbage, fresh mushrooms, leeks and celery
- 1/2 cup dried shiitake mushrooms
- 1/4 cup dried wakame seaweed
- 1 tbsp peppercorns
- 1 - 2 tbsp ground turmeric (use less for a milder taste)
- 1 tbsp coconut aminos,
- A bunch of fresh corriander, or other herb of your choice
- (optional) 1/4 cup nutritional yeast flakes, for extra flavor and vitamins

Instructions:

Simply add everything to a large pot. Bring to a boil then simmer, with the lid on, for about an hour.

Once everything has been cooked down, strain the liquid into a large bowl. Serve immediately with some fresh herbs, for decoration or cool for later. It also freezes well.

Mushroom Broth

Ingredients:

- 1/4 cup olive oil, optional
- 1 1/2 pounds white mushrooms, finely chopped
- Reserved Portobello mushroom stems, brushed clean
- 1/2 Spanish onion, coarsely chopped
- 2 teaspoons chopped garlic
- 2 cups dry white wine
- 1/2 cup soy sauce
- 1/2 cup dried mushrooms, such as porcini or shiitake
- Pinch of salt
- 1/2 teaspoon herbes de Provence or thyme

Directions:

Step 1
In a large non-reactive saucepan, heat the vegetable oil over moderately high heat. Add the white mushrooms, Portobello stems, onion and garlic and cook, stirring, until the mushrooms release their liquid, about 5 minutes.

Step 2
Add the wine, soy sauce, dried mushrooms, salt, herbes de Provence and 6 cups of water and bring to a boil. Cover, reduce the heat to moderate and simmer until the liquid is reduced to about 4 cups, about 1 hour.

Step 3
Pour the broth through a fine strainer into a heat-proof bowl. Strain again, leaving any particles at the bottom of the bowl.

Can be made ahead and stored in the refrigerator up to 4 days.

Turmeric Broth

Ingredients:

- 1–2 tablespoons olive oil (or ghee), optional
- 1 onion- diced
- 1 tablespoons fresh ginger, grated or finely minced
- 4–5 garlic cloves- grated or finely minced
- 1–2 teaspoons turmeric powder or 2–3 teaspoons fresh turmeric, finely grated
- ¼ teaspoon mustard seed (optional)
- 1 teaspoon cumin
- 1 teaspoon coriander
- ¾ – 1 teaspoon sea salt
- 4 cups water
- 4 cups veggie stock
- ¼ teaspoon cayenne, or more to taste
- Squeeze of lime juice or lemon juice (to taste) or 1-2 teaspoons apple cider vinegar (to taste)

Instructions:

Simply add everything to a large pot. Bring to a boil then simmer, with the lid on, for about an hour.

Once everything has been cooked down, strain the liquid into a large bowl.

Bielers Broth

According to Sally Fallon in her book Nourishing Traditions, Dr. Bieler felt that this combination of vegetables was ideal for restoring acid-alkaline and sodium-potassium balance to organs and glands, especially the sodium-loving adrenal glands which suffer under stress. The broth is also supportive for liver function.

Bieler's broth is highly recommended for those under stress or suffering from stress-related conditions.

Ingredients:

- 4 medium zucchini, ends discarded and zucchini sliced into rounds
- 1 pound string beans, ends trimmed
- 2 stalks celery, chopped
- 1-2 bunches parsley (flat-leaf or curly), tough stems removed (you can freeze the stems for stock making)
- 1 sprig each of thyme, rosemary and tarragon
- 4 cups water

Instructions:

Place all ingredients in a pot and bring to a boil. Skim any foam on the surface, lower the heat and simmer, covered until the vegetables are tender, about 15 minutes.

Puree soup in the pot with a handheld blender or in a blender in batches.

Eat warm.

Herbal Broth

Ingredients:

- 2 onions
- 1 head of garlic sliced in half
- 3 carrots
- 4 large celery sticks
- 1 tablespoon pink peppercorns
- small handful fresh parsley
- small handful fresh thyme
- small handful fresh sage

- 3 bay leaves
- 2 cups shiitake mushrooms
- 1/3 cup astragalus root, slices or chopped
- 1 small piece turmeric sliced in half
- 3 inch piece of ginger root sliced thin
- 2-3 pieces kombu seaweed 5 inches in length
- 4 quarts water
- 2 tablespoons extra virgin olive oil, optional

Instructions:

Method 1 (quicker):

- Scrub vegetables clean, cut the carrots and celery into small chunks, halve the onions, slice the garlic bulb in half, slice mushrooms thin.
- Add all ingredients to stock pot and cover with 4 quarts water. Cover, bring to a boil, slide lid half off, and simmer for 1 hour.
- Remove from stove top, let cool, strain through a sieve into a second large pot.

Method 2 (more flavor):

- Peel and dice onions, chop the carrots and celery into small pieces, peel and slice the garlic cloves, slice mushrooms thin.
- Add a splash of extra virgin olive oil to the stock pot, then cook onions, carrots, celery, garlic, mushrooms until softened.
- Add all other ingredients to stock pot and cover with 4 quarts water. Cover, bring to a boil, slide lid half off, and simmer for 1 hour.
- Remove from stove top, let cool, strain through a sieve into a second large pot.

Broth From Scraps

Ingredients:

Throughout the week as you are prepping your meals, smoothies and juices save the cut off pieces and scraps from all of your vegetables in a container in the fridge; potato peels, tomatoes, leathery onion skins, celery and carrot ends, woody mushroom stems, stems and twigs of herbs, zucchini and squash, juice pulp, etc. Keep adding to the scrap bowl until you have enough to make broth.

If after 3 or 4 days you don't have enough scraps, you aren't eating enough vegetables for a plant predominant diet. Two people should have enough scraps in a few days to make a pint of broth and four people should have enough to make a quart of broth every few days.

Directions:

- Put your scraps in a pot and add a few bay leaves and spices. Cover with water 1 ½" over the top of the scraps and bring to a boil.
- Simmer for 30 minutes.
- Cool and strain through a mesh strainer.
- Store in pint or quart jars in the fridge for a week or in the freezer for up to 6 months.

Use this broth to add flavor to your plant based recipes; soup bases, replace water with this broth in rice and beans, use for sauteeing veggies instead of oil. You can freeze in ice cube trays and use a few cubes for sautéing.

Note: Do not use the dried papery skins of onions and garlic, eggplant or artichokes, they make broths taste bitter.

Soups

Our ancestors made soups and stews out of necessity to use what little food they had go a long way. No two pots were ever the same, they used vegetables, greens, roots, herbs and spices and left over meat and bones, if they had it. It warmed them in cold weather, it could feed a lot of people and the cooking broke down the fiber and extracted the nutrients out of the veggies, meat and bones making it nourishing and easy to digest.

Digestive Enzymes

Digestive enzymes are substances secreted by the salivary glands and cells lining the stomach, pancreas, and small intestine to aid in the breakdown of food. Digestive juices require hydration so make sure that you drink water throughout the day.

Digestive enzymes are released both in anticipation of eating, when we first smell and taste food, as well as throughout the digestive process. Some foods have naturally occurring digestive enzymes that contribute to the breakdown of certain specific nutrients.

A variety of foods, especially tropical fruits and fermented vegetables, are naturally high in digestive enzymes that might speed up the digestion of certain nutrients. It's best to consume them raw since heat can lessen or destroy these plant enzymes. All raw food has the enzymes they need to break themselves down.

The more cooked and processed food you eat the more likely you will need to supplement with digestive enzymes.

HCL

Estimates suggest that 1/2 to 3/4 of Americans struggle with having too little stomach acid and continually taking things to reduce stomach acid can make the problem worse.

For good digestion, you need sufficient hydrochloric acid (HCl) and digestive enzyme activity in the gut. These both serve the important function of breaking down food proteins, which prevents the immune system from targeting them and causing symptoms.

HCl is naturally present in the stomach and is vital for digestion of proteins. Low HCl symptoms include:

- Not feeling well after eating meat
- Feeling like meat sits in your stomach too long
- Feeling like you ate a brick
- Acid reflux
- Constipation
- Flatulence
- Colitis

It may sound contrary that low stomach acid can cause acid reflux. In fact, many people with acid reflux-like symptoms are mistakenly prescribed acid-blockers intended to cut stomach acid, when in fact it's low stomach acid causing the problem, the low stomach acid results in undigested food becoming rancid and moving back up the esophagus to cause the pain and burning sensation. What these people need is additional HCl to improve digestion.

Acidity in the stomach is not to be confused with alkalinity of the blood. Hydrochloric acid is the only acid the body produces. All other acids are by-products of metabolism and are eliminated as soon as possible.

Besides absorption, stomach acid is suppose to destroy all

harmful organisms, pathogenic bacteria, parasites, their eggs, and fungi that enter the body through the mouth. If stomach acid is insufficient there is no barrier against parasites. No one can be completely healthy without normal levels of hydrochloric acid.

The natural level of hydrochloric acid decreases as we age, especially after 40. That is when most people begin to get gray hair as a result of nutritional deficiencies caused by lowered stomach acid. People over 65 years old usually have a hard time with protein digestion and trace mineral absorption because of low secretion of stomach hydrochloric acid. This can be confirmed by a comprehensive stool and digestive analysis, and hair mineral analysis. If stomach acid deficiency is the problem, appropriate digestive aids (e.g., herbal bitters, apple cider vinegar, citric acid, betaine, and pepsin HCL, etc.) can be taken with most supplements based on the degree of hypoacidity.

If you have low stomach acid you need to add an HCL supplement midway through your meals.

Raw apple cider vinegar helps to make your stomach more acidic to aid digestion. Sip a teaspoon in a little water before your meal, or add it to your salad dressing. A little sip of pickle juice will help with indigestion, but use caution as white vinegar isn't ideal.

Research suggests indigenous people had stronger stomach acid than we do now and they had much stronger teeth, jaws and jaw muscles to chew tougher plant food, and chew them longer.

Soaking Grains and Nuts for Better Digestion

Phytic acid (an organic acid in which phosphorus is bound) is present in all grains in the outer layer or bran. Untreated phytic acid can combine with calcium, magnesium, copper, iron and especially zinc in the intestinal tract and block their absorption. Soaking or fermenting or sprouting grains allows enzymes, lactobacilli and other helpful organisms to break down and neutralize phytic acid. A diet high in unfermented whole grains, particularly high-gluten grains like wheat, puts an enormous strain on the whole digestive system.

Animals have a different digestive system which is much more acidic enabling them to eat raw grains. But humans need to soak grains before eating them.

Soaking, fermenting or sprouting grains also neutralizes enzyme inhibitors, present in all seeds, and encourages the production of numerous beneficial enzymes. The action of these enzymes also increases the amounts of many vitamins, especially B vitamins. Enzyme inhibitors are part of the seed machinery and serve a purpose. But these inhibitors are out of place in our bodies. They could stop our own enzymes from working. Roasting seeds also neutralizes enzyme inhibitors, but does not provide the enhanced benefits of soaking, fermenting or sprouting.

CHAPTER 15

Divine Detoxification

The Divine Feminine is a sacred energy,
It does not manifest in toxic, polluted environments.

Detoxification occurs on many levels. Physically, this process can help clear congestion, illnesses, and disease potential. Cleansing our minds of negative thought patterns is essential to physical health. Emotionally, detoxification helps us uncover hidden frustrations, anger, resentments, or fear, and replace them with forgiveness, love, joy, and hope. On a spiritual level, many people experience new clarity or an enhancement of their purpose of life during cleansing processes.

Diet is not the key to spiritual life, but it is a positive helping factor that assists in opening the door to communion with the Divine.

- Fasting speeds up spiritual progress.
- Fasting can change hearts and minds.
- Fasting gives you confidence to know that your spirit can master appetite.

- A diet changes the way you look. A fast changes the way you see.
- You can fast for a particular purpose, healing, a specific need or for deeper spiritual awareness.
- You may find you more clearly hear the voice of the spirit inside you.
- Fasting does something that cannot be explained with human language.
- You may experience a sense profound inner peace.

You become aware of just how habitual the act of eating has become. Many of us do not eat for hunger, we eat for pleasure. Absence of constant pleasure exposes you to emotions you mask with your habits, and you are finally exposed to who you really are. This is where the healing process starts, physically, emotionally, and spiritually.

Physical Detoxification

Every Divine Feminine's health and well-being depends on how well her body removes and purges toxins. With exposure to environmental toxins, toxic body care products and processed foods, most of us are in desperate need of a serious detox!

If you are eating a diet high in processed foods, you are putting the health of your liver at risk as these foods basically work against liver health. Hydrogenated oils, refined sugar, convenience foods and lunch meats are notoriously toxic to your system.

Detoxification is the elimination of potential toxic substances from the body. The aim of detoxification is to eliminate toxins and cleanse the body. Our bodies have a natural detoxification system and under optimal circumstances it can detoxify on its own without outside assistance. Though you may be seemingly "healthy", most of us are holding onto toxins, in our gut and our vital organs due to years of not eating the right food and an erratic lifestyle, not allowing our natural detoxification pathways to function properly.

If after 3 to 4 days of fasting you have bad breath, offensive body odor or bodily discharges, this is an indication your system is filled up with decayed substances which have accumulated inside you, from what you have eaten.

Our Ancestors

When our ancestors naturally ate with the seasons nature provided what they needed in each season, to include nourishment, hydration, detoxification and rest.

- Fall provided root vegetables that had starch to keep them warm and put on extra weight as reserved energy they may need when food was more scarce in winter months. The root vegetables overwintered in the ground giving them fresh food into the winter.
- Winter slowed down the animals making it easier to track and hunt them for food. The cold weather kept the meat from spoiling so quickly. The meat took longer to digest keeping their bellies full and the fat kept them warm and gave them energy. They used the hides and fur for protection from the cold. They wasted no part of the animals who sacrificed their lives for them. Winter days were short and the nights were long giving them much needed rest, allowing their bodies to heal and repair while sleeping.
- Spring brought fresh food, sprouting greens and berries for much needed vitamins, minerals, antioxidants and natural detoxification.
- Summer was plentiful with one fruit after the next offering delicious juiciness to keep them hydrated and

provide fiber, vitamins and minerals and liquid sunshine for vibrant health.

- Our ancestors grazed and ate when they were hungry when food was plentiful. They may have eaten once a day or every other day when food was more scarce.

When our bodies are not digesting food they go into detoxification and healing mode. Their lifestyle was automatically set up with intermittent fasting giving their bodies a chance to rest, heal, repair and detoxify themselves rather than constantly eating and digesting as we do today.

Our Toxic World

We live in an unprecedented toxic world where food is plentiful year round and we are constantly eating. Heavy metals are ubiquitous, they are in our water, in our food, in our soil and in our air. Man made chemicals are in our home cleaning and laundry products, our lotions, soaps, shampoos and cosmetics. They are in our lawns, parks and schools.

Did you know that you inherit your mother's toxic load while in the womb? The new born children now have more toxins in them than their mothers. This is one of the reasons generations are becoming sicker and sicker.

Even when you think you are making Divine Feminine healthy choices detoxing is an absolute critical part of maintaining a healthy lifestyle. Detox is short for "detoxification", it's a term used to describe the natural process of purging that takes place within our bodies. The detox process neutralizes toxic waste by absorption or chemically transforming it into a relatively harmless compound and eliminating it from the body via stool, urine, preparation and breath.

Signs You Need to Detox:

- You wake up in the morning with a white coating on your tongue, this is not normal, your tongue should be beautiful pink. A white coating indicates candida albicans/yeast overgrowth, caused by an imbalance in internal body chemistry.
- You regularly wake up tired even though you get plenty of sleep. When you are healthy you wake up energized with a bounce in your step without the need for caffeine to get you going. Having to drag yourself out of bed is a sign that something is off.
- Chronic under eye bags and puffiness may indicate liver congestion, dehydration, lack of sleep, inadequate nutrients, etc. Regardless of the cause, the reality is that they are indicative of poor health and should be addressed sooner rather than later.
- A healthy liver equals healthy skin. If you're struggling with skin issues, chances are your liver is congested. Skin issues can range from acne to dryness, rosacea, psoriasis, redness, itchiness, eczema, etc.
- If you have any digestive issues at all, even if it's just gas, something's off and needs to be addressed. If you regularly have stomach issues, cramps, gas, bloating, IBS, constipation or diarrhea, this is not normal and most likely means you are ingesting foods that your body is hypersensitive to, usually stemming from an unhealthy gut.
- If you have a hard bulging stomach this is an indication you have a lot of old hard fecal matter in your intestines. It is normal to have a few pounds of fecal matter at any given time but with a slow elimination system you can build up to 30 lbs of deadly toxic waste in your intestines absorbing

into your blood steam, making you sick in ways you don't realize are related to this problem.

- Heavy metal toxicity can manifest in many ways. In adults, symptoms can be as varied as memory loss, lack of concentration, unexplained headaches, irritability, depression, nausea, constipation, high blood pressure, joint and muscle pain, numbness and pain in the extremities, fatigue and decreased sex drive. In children, symptoms can include learning disabilities, ADHD, lower IQ, behavioral problems, and decreased bone and muscle growth.

Note: When you undertake any kind of cleanse or detox you may actually feel worse before you feel better, since bacteria releases toxins. Ride it out for a few days and see what happens before giving up. You may need to detox more slowly if you feel ill. As soon as you put food in your mouth your detox slows down or stops, depending on how much you eat. You can eat a little to slow down the process without completely stopping and giving up. Detoxing quickly isn't any better than a slow detox.

There are four main pathways of toxic elimination in the body; perspiration, breath, urine and defecation. To successfully excrete toxins from the body while on a cleanse you have to open up each pathway.

Detoxing provides a way to keep the excess waste in your body on the move. Routine detox helps your body purge itself of these toxic residues, enhancing the function of your liver, kidney and colon.

When you have a clean colon and liver, the rate at which these toxins are re-introduced to your body decreases significantly.

Begin Your Detox

The first thing you have to do is stop putting the crap in your body that you will need to clean out and eliminate, before it causes you harm.

The next thing to know is that during a fast your body will burn up stored fat as energy. Most of us have plenty of that. You will not starve. You will not die.

2 Week Pre-Detox:

Your chosen detox plan will be much more effective and easier on your body if you first eliminate the following to clear out accumulated debris which will open the detox pathways.

- Minimize or eliminate processed food, sugar, white flour and fried food. Simply eliminating these foods is the first step to a healthier lifestyle of effective detox.
- Mono meals, eating only one food per meal until satisfied, is easy and quick to digest to assist in natural detoxification.
- Eliminating meat during a detox frees up time and energy. Cooked meat is the hardest thing for the digestive system to break down and eliminate.
- Pasteurized and homogenized dairy is acidic and mucus forming. It is best to eliminate dairy products for an effective detox.
- Increase water intake to flush out toxins through the urine, perspiration and bowel movements.
- Increase fiber intake to scrub intestines and move out old fecal matter and absorb loosened toxins.
- If constipation has been a problem for you, herbal laxatives, aloe vera, castor oil, coffee enemas and colonics can be very helpful in moving out built up waste in the

intestines. If you have been ill colonic treatments will speed up the detox and recovery.

Constipation

Research over the last hundred years shows that bowel toxins actually exist. Not only do they exist, but they have a tremendous negative impact on mental and physical well-being. Toxins usually come from a process called intestinal toxemia, an overgrowth of putrefactive intestinal bacteria in the small and large intestine. These toxins are then absorbed into the blood stream and from there affect both our mental and physical functioning. Intestinal toxemia is predominantly caused by an excessively high animal protein diet. Overeating, eating late at night, and/or a slowing of bowel eliminative function directly contribute to it. Constipation also contributes a lot to this bowel toxemia.

Fasting is one of the best and quickest treatments for bowel toxicity. The fasting process allows the bowels to rest and the inflammation to subside. If there are no proteins on which to feed, the putrefactive bacteria will also diminish. For those who do not want to fast, a low-protein diet (20-30 grams of protein per day), along with a high-complex-carbohydrate, 80%raw-food diet, is a slower but effective cure.

The body's first line of defense is a healthy colon. Sluggish functions of this organ can rapidly produce widespread toxicity and autointoxication, making colon cleansing one of the most important parts of the detoxification process. When you become constipated you quickly reabsorb toxins, poisons, chemicals and hormones. You also absorb water from your colon which makes your stool harder, dryer and larger. This makes you feel tied and sluggish and gives you stomach aches, gas, headaches and hemorrhoids.

Before beginning any detox plan you have to clean out your

colon to open up your biggest elimination pathway to rid your body of old fecal matter, parasites, yeasts and bacteria, toxins and poisons.

Most people are shocked to learn an average person carries 5 to 10 pounds of fecal matter, dead microorganisms, undigested food remnants, slime, fermentation byproducts and other foul material. A chronically constipated person can have 20 pounds or more of compacted fecal matter in their gut.

Colon Cleanses

Sea Salt Water Flush for Constipation

Intake of salt water increases your bowel movements and helps expel various toxins, bacteria, and accumulated feces from your colon. The sodium in the salt pulls water from your tissues into your intestines. Salt water colon cleansing is also comparatively safe and ensures that your body doesn't lose too many electrolytes.

Ingredients:

- 2 teaspoons of sea salt
- glass jar with a lid
- 1 liter of hot filtered water
- 2 tablespoons of fresh lemon juice (for taste)

Directions:

- Heat up your water but not to boiling.
- Add your ingredients into the jar and put the lid on. Shake it vigorously to fully dissolve the salt. Make sure no granules are visible. Let it cool down a bit.
- Drink the warm mixture quickly, within a few minutes if possible (under 5 minutes is the goal).

- Lay down on your side and massage your belly on one side, then repeat on the other side. Within a short time after finishing the mixture you should start to feel the urge to go to the bathroom.
- Once you feel you can no longer hold out, go to the bathroom. You might have to go more than one time, sometimes needing to use the bathroom for several hours before you're fully "cleansed" and your colon is emptied. It is best to do this in the morning.

Vitamin C Flush

Not only does the vitamin C flush move your bowls if you are constipated, it flushes out parasites and bugs that may be living in your intestines. The flush happens so quickly they don't have time to burrow in and hide. A word of warning, if you have such things in you they will come out alive and you could see them swimming in the toilet.

A Vitamin C Flush is one of the easiest and quickest detoxification methods. It's simply introducing high amounts of vitamin C into the body at regular intervals until the intestines flush themselves with a watery stool. Our body absorbs the vitamin C it needs and when the tissues are saturated your body flushes out the excess.

Like any detoxification program, afterwards the body feels refreshed and rejuvenated. The benefits of an ascorbic acid flush do not end there. It is also a way to boost the body's vitamin C stores and absorption rate. Each time a cleansing flush is done, the body needs less of the nutrient to reach its ideal level. In fact, doing an ascorbic acid flush will tell you exactly how much vitamin C your unique body needs.

Seventy-five percent of the amount of Vitamin C required to flush our you system, is your own personal recommended daily intake for optimal health.

How To Do A Vitamin C Flush

It is important to use ascorbic acid powder or buffered ascorbic acid powder. The buffered version is combined with a buffer mineral such as calcium, magnesium, zinc, etc. or a combination of all three that is gentler on your stomach and intestines, but may be less effective. For maximum effectiveness stick to regular ascorbic acid powder, if you can tolerate it.

Take a spoonful in a half-glass of filtered/purified water every twenty to thirty minutes, keeping track of the total spoonfuls of ascorbic acid taken. Do this until you have a soupy, watery stool.

Once the Vitamin C Flush is completed, you can continue taking smaller doses of ascorbic acid every four hours for the next couple days, trying to maintain a thicker, tapioca-like stool. If diarrhea occurs again, lower the dosage. This can be done for a more thorough detoxification, but is not required.

To optimize the Vitamin C Flush, start in the morning on an empty stomach. Expect to cleanse for two to four hours, although for some people, more time is needed. Be sure to drink adequate water during the flush.

A Vitamin C Flush can be done as often as once a month or once every four months.

The healthier your body is, the less vitamin C you will require. So, the more vitamin C it takes to flush your system the more your body NEEDS vitamin C.

Bentonite Clay

The name of the clay stems from the town, Fort Beonton, Montana, where today much of the supply is still harvested. The other name that bentonite clay is typically given, Montmorillonite clay, stems from the region of France called Montmorillon, where the clay was first discovered.

Bentonite Clay is Mother Nature's pharmacy. It is volcanic ash with all the impurities burned out leaving pure trace minerals. Clay is a nano crystal of highly charged electromagnetic energy from the thermodynamic heat of a volcano. It can not be duplicated in a laboratory. Only Mother Nature can make clay.

Bentonite clay stems back far in history as a traditional healing method for protecting the body from disease. It has been reported that several traditional cultures living in regions of the Andes, Central Africa and Australia have applied and consumed volcanic clays in numerous ways for centuries. The medicine men of many aboriginal tribes have long used clay as part of their healing treatments. There is a long recorded history of animals in the wild instinctually seeking and eating clay to heal themselves.

Bentonite Clay's strength lies in its ability to adsorb and suck into itself toxins, chemicals, viruses, molds, and the bad bacteria, hold them captive within the molecule and carry them out of the body.

Another use for bentonite clay, is adsorption of radiation, such as the Fukushima nuclear disaster in Japan. Not only does bentonite clay adsorb radiation from nuclear fallout, it also adsorbs any kind of radiation, to include xrays and EMF's from cell phones and wifi's.

Internal Cleanse: Taken orally, bentonite clay is used to detoxify the digestive system, eliminate intestinal parasites, strengthen the immune system, and fight free radicals. It also helps remove heavy metals from the body and assists in the process of liver detoxification.

Internal Benefits: acid reflux/heartburn, allergies/hay fever, celiacs disease, constipation, diarrhea/dysentery, diverticulitis, detox/heavy metals, food poisoning, h-pylori, hiatel hernia, irritable bowel syndrom (IBS), Crohn's Disease, menstrual cramps, parasites, Roto Virus, stomach ache/stomach flu, diabetes, ulcers.

- When starting the clay internally, go slow!
- Start with 1/3 tsp daily and drink plenty of water.
- During the 2nd week, take 2/3 tsp, working your way up to 1 tsp of clay a day.
- This will minimize the "healing crisis" your body will experience as the clay cleans and detoxes.

Letting the mixture sit overnight, and allowing the sediment to settle and drinking just the clay water from the top of the mixture in the morning is another gentle approach.

Castor Oil

Castor oil is a powerful laxative that can quicken and increase your bowel movements. The ricinoleic acid present in castor oil has potential laxative effects. It could help in cleansing your colon by expelling the unwanted toxins from your body.

- 1-2 tablespoons of castor oil
- 1-2 tablespoons of orange or lemon juice (unsweetened)

Directions:

- Mix castor oil and the orange or lemon juice in equal amounts.
- Drink this on an empty stomach, early in the morning.
- After every 15-30 minutes, drink a glass of hot water until you have emptied your bowels at least 2 to 3 times.

Probiotics After Colon Cleanse

Adding lactobacillus acidophilus (normal large intestine bacteria) culture to the system helps to re-populate the small and large intestine with healthy bacteria, therefore diminishing putrefactive(abnormal) bacteria. Exercise also helps to stimulate the digestive system. Although many will respond to these basic aids to digestion, in the short run one may need some digestive enzymes and/or digestion-stimulating herbs to help rest and rebuild the digestive power that has been weakened after long years of abuse.

Fasting

Fasting is the first principle of medicine. Fasting accelerates the healing process and allows the body to recover from disease in a short time.

Nature teaches us there is but one disease, basically caused by overeating and eating the wrong things. What ever name man my put to it, can be cured by one remedy; withholding from the body the substances which normally bring about the diseases. Studies find that fasting for 72 hours can regenerate the entire immune system.

Some people don't feel well when they fast or miss a meal, they may get light headed, nauseous or dizzy, thinking they have low blood sugar, but studies have shown this is not usually the case. The discomfort most people feel when they don't eat is actually the body beginning to detox. The more toxins you have in you, the worse you will feel once they are stirred up and your body begins eliminating them. In other words, the worse you feel when you go without eating, the more toxic you are.

Your body is very intelligent, it knows how to heal and repair itself. Your body's job is to stay alive, it wants to live and it knows how to prioritize which things to heal first and what can wait. It will heal what is the most life threatening first, not necessarily what you want healed first.

Your body has to digest and eliminate the food you put in your mouth. Digestion is high on the priority list of bodily functions.

If it can't digest and eliminate the food, it will rot and putrefy inside of you and you will die. A lot of blood flow and energy goes to digesting food. Once digestion is completed the body begins healing and detoxing. As soon as you put food in your mouth, healing and detoxing stops and the attention goes back to digestion.

If you are continually eating you are continually digesting, therefore not spending enough time healing and repairing. For this reason, eating 2 or 3 meals a day is better than continually grazing or snacking between meals.

Intermittent Fasting

"Hunger is the first element of self-discipline. If you can control what you eat and drink, you can control everything else.

Fasting allows the body to rest from the hard work of digestion. Intermittent fasting gives your body time to heal and repair in between meals without long periods of starving yourself.

Intermittent fasting is when you allow yourself to eat only during a specified window of time each day. It usually involves fasting for a certain number of hours or even days that are spaced out during the week, and there's no "right" way to do this. The best way is what works for you and fits into your schedule.

One plan is 16:8, you only eat during eight hours of the day, usually eating just two meals a day. You can technically choose when you want your eight-hour period to be, but most people tend to stop eating at a certain time in the evening, like 6 p.m., and then wait to eat again 16 hours later (in this case, it would be at 10 a.m.). That way, you are sleeping for part of your fast instead of sitting around, thinking about the food you're not eating for a good part of the day.

Intermittent fasting lowers insulin levels and improves insulin sensitivity, lowers blood pressure and decreases appetite. Intermittent fasting has also been linked to increased neuroplasticity, or the brain's ability to form new synaptic connections and fight injury.

Liquid Fasting

Stop eating and drink water, herbs (greens) and juice. A liquid fast is beneficial to take the stress off of the digestive system by "predigesting" your food in a blender or juicer and making soups, broths and teas. This is easier for most people to do than a severe water fast.

Green Smoothies: Green smoothies include a number of green vegetables containing chlorophyll, which helps in detoxification and getting rid of heavy metals like those found in pesticides and industrial pollutants.

- Start your day with this green smoothie to provide energy and boost metabolism.
- Put one cup of kale (coarsely chopped). If you do not have kale, then use collard greens.
- one green apple (coarsely chopped)
- one ripe banana
- one-half cup of fresh parsley leaves or cilantro in a blender

Blend the ingredients with about two or two and one-half cups of water. Start by drinking one cup of this smoothie daily. Gradually increase the dosage to three to four cups a day for at least three weeks.

Green Smoothie Recipes

The whole point of green smoothies is to consume more greens. Any leafy greens can be used. They are especially beneficial for those with digestive and dental issues.

A high powered blender, such as a VitaMix, is needed for a smooth consistency, rather than chunky. Blending the fruits, greens and vegetables in this way "pre-digests" the food for much easier digestion. It is easier to drink a green smoothie than chew a big salad.

Green smoothies can be sweet or savory. For beginners and children sweet smoothies using mild flavored greens such as romaine and red leaf lettuce with added fruit are sweetly favored and well received. When called for I prefer using frozen bananas, fresh bananas feel slimy when blended at high speed, but you can use either. When bananas become too ripe for me to eat I peel them, break them in half, put them in a baggie and freeze them to use in smoothies.

Savory smoothies using kale, chard and spinach can include onions, garlic, lemon, lime, basil, cilantro, parsley, dill, mint, hot and bell peppers, tomatoes, and avocados. A pinch of sea salt improves the taste for those coming off a salty standard American diet. And a little heat adds interest and some pizzaz for the taste buds. Flavor your smoothies to your hearts content.

Lemon Jalapeno Fresca

- ½ lemon, juiced
- 4 Roma tomatoes
- 5 kale leaves
- ½ inch jalapeno pepper
- 1 small garlic clove
- 2 cups water

Place all ingredients in a high power blender and blend on high until smooth.

Tomato Dill

- 5 kale leaves
- ½ bunch fresh dill
- ½ lime, juiced
- 3 garlic cloves
- 1/4 cup sun dried tomatoes
- 2 cups water

Place all ingredients in a high power blender and blend on high until smooth.

Apple Banana

- 2 handfuls spinach leaves
- 4 apples, peeled
- ½ lime, juiced
- 1 banana, frozen
- 2 cups water

Place all ingredients in a high power blender and blend on high until smooth.

Strawberry Banana

- 1 Cup strawberries, fresh or frozen
- 1 - 2 bananas, frozen
- 1 bunch romaine lettuce
- 2 cups water

Place all ingredients in a high power blender and blend on high until smooth.

Raw Juice Fasting

Unless you are doing a one-day juice cleanse, you will want to prepare your body for your juice fast. If you are doing two, three day or more cleanse, you will want to consider the recommendations below. If you jump right into the cleanse from an unhealthy diet, also known as SAD (standard American diet), you could feel quite sick from the detox side effects and not want to continue or even attempt it again.

The week before a juice fast:

- Transition unhealthy meals and junk food out of your diet and replace them with more raw organic vegetables and fruit making about 75 to 80 percent of your diet raw and whole foods.
- Eat smaller portions than usual, eating only enough to satisfy your hunger.
- Incorporate regular, non-strenuous exercise into your routine.
- Make sure you are drinking enough clean water, which is key to flushing out toxins.

Raw fruit and vegetable juices, such as that of apples, carrots, grapefruits, spinach, blueberries, oranges, cucumbers, beets, and lettuce, are highly beneficial for nourishing your body as well as removing harmful toxins. They are a rich source of vitamins, minerals, dietary fiber and many other biologically active compounds.

Many of these phytochemicals stimulate the immune system, hormone metabolism, reduce blood pressure and even regulate detoxification enzymes of the body.

Juices extracted from green vegetables are particularly

beneficial because they contain chlorophyll, which alkalizes the body and aids in the removal of cancer-related toxins.

Juices are more easily digested by the body since the indigestible fibers of vegetables and fruits are removed and the nutrients are also more easily available to the body in comparison to whole vegetables and fruits.

You can simply drink a glass of raw fruit or vegetable juice two or three times a day or replace one meal daily with fresh juices on a regular basis. For a juice fast, drink six to eight glasses of fresh fruit and vegetable juices daily for a few days.

If you are juicing fruit it is advisable to dilute the juice with water to avoid consuming too much sugar in a short time. Always drink water between juices during the day.

In addition to juice from a single fruit or vegetable, you can create a juice blend by juicing five carrots, four celery stalks, one beet, one small apple, one small cucumber, and half a lemon.

For better absorption of the dense nutrients, drink the juice slowly rather than quickly gulping it down.

During the juice cleanse:

- Drink warm lemon water. It's an incredible liver stimulant and it helps begin the cleansing process before you even take a sip of that first juice. Once getting into the habit of it during your cleanse, you might find that it is something that you want to continue to do post-cleanse. In addition to drinking your allotment of water, you can also include herbal tea into your cleanse plan.
- Choose and prepare your produce wisely whether you are making your juices at home or buying them from a juice bar.
- Choose organic vegetables, herbs and fruit whenever possible. A good rule of thumb is to have green juice make up at least half of your juice consumption.

- Wash everything well. Even if it is organic, it still can have undesirable organisms or other contaminants on it.
- Aim to drink a juice every 2 to 2.5 hours. 6 to 8 juices a day might sound like a lot but if you space your juices out over 12 hours, your body will thank you.

Dry Brush: This probably sounds crazy since juicing is all about cleaning you internally but dry brushing your skin daily during your cleanse will help get rid of dead skin and open your pores for the elimination process.

Exercise Lightly: Listen to your body. Your energy levels can change and be a bit unpredictable during a cleanse so you may want to limit yourself to light exercise like walks, yoga, and stretching.

Focusing on Relaxing: Allow your body and mind to relax. Meditate every day or begin a journal where you can write about your day and how you're feeling. Get plenty of rest and take naps if possible.

Breaking the juice cleanse

End your cleanse when you feel the time is right. After you finish your cleanse, celebrate what you've accomplished. Every day that you juiced, you nourished your body with around 20 pounds of nutrients. That's something to applaud yourself for!

Now is a great time to think about how you want to incorporate what you've learned into your daily regimen. Maybe you will want to swap one meal a day with vegetable juice? Or maybe two?

The day after your cleanse you're going to want to ease into solid foods. I have found one of the best ways to come off a cleanse is to drink smoothies and eat small pieces of juicy, watery fruit.

In the days following a cleanse, you have the opportunity to identify any food sensitivities. If you suspect you are allergic to something, systematically add it to your diet and see if it's a trigger for you.

I like doing juice cleanses not only to periodically deep clean, but to really focus on myself and check in with my body to make sure I'm understanding what it needs. I encourage you to try a juice cleanse, and while they may seem difficult at first, if you stick to it, you won't believe how amazing you will feel!

Fasting is safe and can be beneficial for most people, although some people should fast under supervision and some not at all. You should consult a health professional if you are unsure if you should do a juice fast.

Liver Cleanse

There is a strong link between a healthy, fully-functioning liver and your overall health. The liver fulfills hundreds of critical functions including metabolizing carbohydrates and protein, storing vitamins, converting nutrients into energy, and more. When it stops performing these tasks efficiently, then you have a liver problem.

It sifts through every single thing that comes into your body and uses what it can and gets rid of what it can't, so it's important to keep things coming in that your body can use, rather than things it has to filter out because it recognizes them as harmful invaders.

In fact, between filtering your blood, detoxifying chemicals, metabolizing foods and other outside substances, your liver is a vital organ for life and weight loss.

To spot a potential liver problem, you need to be on the lookout for the following symptoms:

- Digestive difficulties
- Diabetes
- Obesity
- Fatigue and lack of energy
- Arthritis

You will notice that each of these issues can hinder your weight loss efforts as well, especially Type 2 diabetes and digestive issues. If you are suffering from any of these symptoms, then it's possible that you're suffering from liver problems.

If you want to remove the buildup of toxins and restore your liver's metabolic capabilities, then you should consider liver detoxification. A liver detox can involve switching to a specific diet (such as avoiding sugar and simple carbohydrates), taking on a juice fast, or using natural supplements such as herbal and homeopathic formulas to cleanse the liver of toxins and chemical buildups.

Your liver has two stages of detoxification, known as Phase 1 and Phase 2. All of these tips will aid in both steps of detoxification without you feeling sick and like someone stole the life out of you in the process. There's no need to go on crazy cleanses. Take care of your body with a whole foods, no junk, and booze-free plant predominant diet, and be sure you exercise and get some fresh air and sun shine whenever you can.

Your liver has to detoxify everything you put in your mouth. Take the load off the liver and eat less, eat organic, drink lots of water and use as little chemical medications as possible.

Optimizing your diet with fresh, plant-based foods is a great place to start. It takes effort, but a liver detox will not only remove the toxins preventing your liver from properly metabolizing your food, it help prevent future liver issues.

Water

Your liver likes to be clean (much like you do!) and what's better than keeping it clean with fresh, alkalizing water? Living water contains natural minerals when it comes from a healthy source (not from chlorinated tap waters), so use spring or well water when you can, or check with your city's water to see if it's environmentally safe (some areas are better than others). Also, use a water filtration system that removes the carbon and chlorine particles when possible. Add a squeeze of lemon to your water to add even more alkalizing and cleansing properties. Lemon and all citrus fruits contain vitamin C and minerals that boost bodily functions and enhance the cleansing process, sweeping out wastes. Flushing your liver is like giving your body a good pre-wash so your blood stays at optimal pH levels. Aim for as many glasses a day as you can or drink caffeine-free herbal tea as a second option.

Too Much Protein

Liver problems stem from two causes: 'overworking' the liver and the buildup of toxins. The two are interconnected in that they both occur from consuming too much protein, too many carbohydrates, trans fats, too much alcohol, lack of exercise and others.

Avoid Chemicals

Not only does your liver process chemicals that enter your body through your mouth, but it also processes chemicals that enter through your nose and skin. Some everyday household products contain toxins that can damage your liver, especially if you come into contact with them regularly. To prevent long-term damage to your liver, opt for organic cleaning products and techniques to clean your home. Avoid using pesticides and herbicides in your yard, or take precautions to avoid inhaling chemical fumes.

If you must use chemicals or aerosols inside the house, to paint for instance, make sure your space is well ventilated. If that's not possible, wear a mask.

Exercise

Some tried-and-true liver-friendly habits include eating a balanced diet, exercising regularly, and protecting yourself from potentially harmful medications, liver diseases, and environmental toxins.

Fruits and Vegetables

Eating healthy food for the liver is one of the best ways to prevent liver damage. Fresh fruits and vegetables contain powerful antioxidants that help the liver do its job and keep it clean. Cruciferous vegetables like broccoli, cabbage, and cauliflower contribute to good liver health, as do high-fiber foods such as apples, brown rice, and strawberries. Garlic and onions provide a number of health benefits.

Juicing

Juicing is like taking a natural nutritional supplement. It is very potent condensed nutrition, especially good for the weak or ill. It is better than a pill or powder as it is raw, whole, easily digestible and can quickly be used by the body.

It can be nearly impossible to eat all of the raw vegetables you need to make your liver cleanse effective. However, by juicing a variety of raw vegetables, you can easily get the 4–5 servings of fresh, organic vegetables you need. Even vegetables that aren't your favorites can be disguised and enjoyed in a fresh vegetable juice!

Turmeric

Turmeric is well-known for its medicinal and healing properties. It also detoxifies your liver, purifies the blood, and is beneficial for lung and colon health too. Plus, it has anti-inflammatory, antioxidant, and anti-cancerous properties.

- Add one teaspoon of turmeric powder, juice from one lemon, a pinch of cayenne pepper, and a little honey (to taste) to one cup of warm water. Drink this once daily for a few days or weeks.
- Alternatively, boil two cups of water, add one-half teaspoon each of turmeric powder and dry ginger powder, and let it simmer for 10 minutes. Then strain the tea and add juice from half a lemon and one tablespoon of pure maple syrup. Drink this daily or a few times a week for a few weeks.

Parasite Cleanse

Parasites are everywhere. We can get them from contaminated food and water (including water in lakes, ponds, and rivers), improperly cooked meat (pork is notorious for containing parasites), contaminated fruits and vegetables, walking barefoot on contaminated soil, and other places. Owning pets and traveling to third world countries can also increase your risk of parasites.

When your immune system is weak, you are more likely to contract a parasite infection. Imbalances in gut bacteria, poor diet, chronic stress, poor sleeping habits, unnecessary use of antibiotics, and other factors can weaken your immune system. This may predispose you to a parasite infection.

Parasites are organisms that can live inside your body and cause illness. They can harm your body in many ways, causing everything from muscle aches to blood infections. There are innumerable parasites that can infect and live in your body. These include bacteria, viruses and worms. If left untreated, parasites can consume the nutrients from the food you eat and produce toxic waste products, which can lead to destruction of body tissues.

Parasites can easily go undetected because they bury themselves in the walls of organs and lining of the intestines trying to guarantee their survival.

The moon cycle and the parasite life cycle are totally in sync. Like so many other things that come out/are more active during the full moon, so do parasites! Literally, from the folds, twists and turns in the lining of the colon. It only makes sense that this is the best time to do a parasite, colon cleanse. Watch the calendar and be ready to do this at least three months in a row to take on the 1) eggs that are being laid, 2) babies that are growing into adults, and 3) adults themselves.

Parasite cleansing is recommended during a Full Moon phase, because the several days before and on the New Moon parasites detach from the walls of the organs and lining of the intestines to breed and to lay eggs. This makes the Full Moon phase the easiest time to get to rid them. **Parasite cleanse start time is 3-4 days before next Full Moon phase.**

Supplements

You can take herbs to help naturally cleanse your body of parasites.

- Take one 500 mg turmeric tablet once daily, and sprinkle turmeric to your food. Turmeric contains an active ingredient called curcumin, a substance that can destroy parasites internally and limit the inflammation caused by extensive tissue damage, says naturopathic physician and co-author of the "Encyclopedia of Natural Medicine," Dr. Michael Murray.

- Take one 500 mg bearberry capsule once daily. The bearberry herb contains a powerful substance called arbutin. It works by dissolving the cellular walls of numerous parasitic bacteria, which can infiltrate your body and cause illness, according to naturopathic physician Dr. Mark Percival.
- Add two to three cloves of garlic to your food or take it in tablet form.When consumed internally, garlic transforms your gastrointestinal tract into a very hostile environment for many parasites. The active ingredients in garlic are ajoene and allicin, both of which can destroy parasites, including one-cell varieties, hookworms and pinworms, according to Dr. Cedric Garland, professor at University of California, San Diego (UCSD) School of Medicine. The recommended dosage for garlic in tablet form is one 500 mg once daily.
- Echinacea is a powerful herb that can stimulate the cells of your immune system to assist in eliminating disease-causing parasites, according to naturopathic physician Dr. Richard Schulze. The recommended dosage for echinacea is one 500 mg tablet once every day, preferably with food.

These are just a few helpful preventative and maintenance herbs. There are also many other herbal formulas specifically for parasite cleanses at health stores. Natural parasite cleanse programs should last 7 to 14 days (or longer, if you suspect a lot of them) to allow the parasites to complete the breeding cycle and the new eggs to hatch and die off. It's not uncommon to have some die-off symptoms during this time. The die-off symptoms are a result from the toxins released as the parasites die, one last attempt they make at trying to live. These symptoms can imitate the flu, but typically show up as a rash.

Also it's good to do a follow-up cleanse to make sure that any egg larva don't remain. After a consecutive three or four month parasite cleanse you should do a parasite cleanse every six months or annually thereafter, as maintenance.

Yeast Cleanse

Candida overgrowth occurs when the balance between candida and the good bacteria is being disturbed. Candida changes into a more aggressive fungal form that spreads and releases over 80 different toxins. These toxins can get anywhere in the body, suppress the immune system and cause a wide variety of health issues all over the body.

The most common causes of candida are antibiotics use, contraceptive pill (birth control pill), high blood sugar issues, and diet high in sugars or processed foods. In many cases, there are less obvious causes of candida such as chronic stress, food allergies you may not be aware of, a weakened immune system, chronic constipation and others. Finding the underlying cause of your issues in most cases is the most important step in order to treat candida overgrowth and other candidiasis related yeast infection issues.

Most candida overgrowth and yeast infections are caused by a strand of yeast called Candida Albicans. A yeast overgrowth can impact liver and kidney function, as well as proper digestion and the health of your skin and mucosal membranes.

Before starting a yeast cleanse find out what causes candida overgrowth in your body. Certain medication, antibiotics, high sugar diet and chronic stress are common causes of candida overgrowth. This is very important, as long as the cause of your candida overgrowth is still present you won't be able to completely heal the candida yeast overgrowth.

Before the candida cleanse has a very effective way to clear existing candida yeast toxins and stored waste you have to do a colon cleanse first. Accumulated waste buildup in the colon is one of the main reasons candida yeasts toxins circulate in the body longer making you feel sick. Removing the toxic waste buildup before the yeast cleanse has shown to make a significant difference in minimizing the candida die off reaction.

Candida Cleanse foods to avoid include simple carbs such as:

- sugars
- refined starches
- peeled white potatoes
- white rice
- processed foods
- sugary beverages
- dairy
- gluten
- white flour, bread, pasta, crackers, breakfast cereal
- alcohol
- mold, blue cheese, Gorgonzola, Brie
- bakers yeast
- foods that are hard to digest such as beans and legumes which haven't been pre-soaked
- common food allergens such as seafood, peanuts.

The best foods for the candida cleanse clean eating; plant based, whole foods:

- fresh greens
- non-starchy veggies such as broccoli, cauliflower
- low sugary fruits such as berries, kiwis or grapefruit.
- avocados, coconut oil or coconut butter
- fresh raw sprouted nuts and seeds

The levels of candida typically go down as a result of limiting candida's preferred fuel source (sugars) coupled with clean eating.

Anti-fungal foods that kill candida should be introduced slowly to your candida cleanse diet so you get the candida yeast cleansing benefits while minimizing a die off reaction.

Common foods that can kill yeast and candida include:

- raw fresh garlic
- ginger
- coconut oil
- cinnamon and others

You can find a complete list of anti-fungal foods on the internet.

There are many good herbal yeast cleanses available at health stores. Ask a clerk to help you understand the differences between them to make the best choice for yourself.

To effectively get yeast overgrowth under control:

- Find the root cause and fix it.
- Stop eating the food that feeds it. You can't kill it and feed it at the same time.
- Eat anti-fungal foods and herbs.
- Eat a whole food plant predominant diet.
- Take an herbal yeast cleanse, colloidal silver and probiotics.
- Always eat more fiber to move out the toxins and die off.

The yeast cleanse salad dressing: raw unpasteurized apple cider vinegar, lemon juice, olive oil, ground cayenne pepper (optional) and himalayan pink salt. Adding hemp seeds and avocado with this salad dressing can turn any veggie salad into a complete meal. Adding pumpkin seeds will add another antifungal candida killing element.

Add More Fiber With All Detoxification Programs

Fiber acts as the scrubbers of the intestines to loosen and remove toxic debris, built up waste and parasites. It also absorbs toxins, hormones and chemicals that are being stirred up as you detox. Without adequate fiber to carry out and eliminate the extra load of toxic waste you could become very ill.

Fiber, found in plant-based foods such as fruits and vegetables, helps with nutrient absorption and removes toxins via stool. Dietary fiber increases the bulk of stool, helps promote regular bowel movements, and reduces the time that waste spends inside the intestines.

Your digestive tract uses probiotics from fiber to nourish your intestines with beneficial bacteria, which helps maintain immune health.

Most people in the United States do not get enough fiber from their diets. According to some estimates, only 5% of the population meet the adequate intake recommendations. If these same people began a detox program without stepping up their fiber they would be very miserable.

According to the Academy of Nutrition and Dietetics, the recommended intake for dietary fiber in a 2,000 calorie diet is:

- 25 grams (g) per day for adult females.
- Women need less fiber after 50 years of age, at around 21 g
- During pregnancy or breast-feeding, women should aim for at least 28 g per day.

Tips for increasing fiber:

- Eat fruits and vegetables with the skins on, as the skins contain lots of fiber
- Add beans or lentils to salads, soups, and side dishes

- Replace white breads and pastas for whole grain versions
- Aim to eat 4.5 cups of vegetables and 4.5 cups of fruit each day
- Add raw nuts, seeds to your daily diet

Flax Seeds:

Flax seeds are rich sources of omega-3 fatty acids. The daily consumption of flax seeds is a sure shot way to cleanse your colon due to the combined bulking effect and laxative effect of its compounds. While the omega-3s are wonderful for your overall health, the seeds also contain antioxidants and fiber that could help increase your bowel movements and flush out the toxins from your body.

- 1 tablespoon of powdered flax seeds
- 1 glass of warm water

Take a tablespoon of ground flax seeds and mix with a glass of warm water. Consume this mixture 30 minutes before you have breakfast and before going to bed.

Note: You can also add some honey for flavor. Drink this mixture twice a day. Keep ground flax seeds in the freezer as they may go rancid very quickly.

Chia Seeds:

The seed is packed with nutrients and delivers a powerful punch of energizing power. The great Aztec warriors used them to provide them with high levels of energy throughout the day and increased stamina. They consumed just one spoonful of chia seeds to sustain them for the entire day. The word "chia" means "strength" in the Mayan language. Chia seeds were also known as the "food for runners" since warriors and runners were able to use the seeds as an energy source to sustain them while running long distances or while in battle.

Among the many reasons why chia seeds are so beneficial include having high amounts of fiber, protein, omega-3 fatty acids, vitamins, and minerals. The most optimal way to get the vitamins and minerals in the seeds is to either soak or grind them. When you soak them, you basically "sprout" them, thus releasing the "enzyme inhibitors" which are used to protect the chia seed.

Just 2 tablespoons of chia seeds give you 40% of your recommended daily fiber. You can add chia seeds to water, juice, smoothies, cereals, baked goods, jams and make chia pudding.

Chia Pudding

- 1/4 cup chia seeds, whole seeds, not ground
- 3/4 cup full fat coconut milk
- 1/2 cup juice or water of your choice
- a splash of vanilla extract (optional)
- a pinch of Himalayan salt

Directions:

- Stir well and allow to chill in the fridge for several hours or overnight.
- Sweeten to taste with your favorite sweetener like honey or pure maple syrup.
- You can top with fruits, coconut flakes and nuts.
- Variation: Serve chia pudding with fruit puree made of frozen pineapple.

Chocolate Chia Pudding

- 1 cup unsweetened vanilla almond milk
- 6 Tablespoons chia seeds

- 1/4 cup maple syrup, honey or sweetener of choice
- 2 Tablespoons cocoa powder
- 1/8 teaspoon salt
- 1 teaspoon vanilla extract
- toppings of choice: fresh berries chocolate chips, nuts

Directions:

Add almond milk, chia seeds, maple syrup, cocoa powder, vanilla and salt into a high powered blender. Start at a low setting on your blender (variable on the Vitamix) and progress to high. Blend until chia seeds are almost undetectable and mixture is smooth, scraping down the sides of the blender with a spatula if needed.

Chia pudding should be thick and ready to enjoy so you can top with your favorite toppings and dive in or if you like your chocolate pudding cold, cover and refrigerate for 3-4 hours to chill before eating.

Whole Oats

The insoluble fiber helps reduce constipation, promotes a full feeling for long periods of time, and may help reduce overall LDL cholesterol.

More than half the fiber in your bowl of oatmeal comes from soluble fiber, specifically beta glucan. During digestion, beta glucan dissolves in water and forms a type of gel. As this gel travels through your digestive system, it grabs onto bile acids and carries them out of your body. Bile acids are primarily made up of cholesterol. To replace the bile acids that left with the beta glucan, your body must pull cholesterol from your blood, which is how it lowers your number.

Whole oats are the uncut, unsteamed, unrolled oat groat. In many cases, whole oats are cut with steel cutters, into two or three pieces, to make steel-cut oats. As they are made from unprocessed, whole grains, whole oats have a round, slightly bulbous texture. Rolled oats, meanwhile, are steel cut oats that have been steamed and rolled flat. They are medium-small in size and cook more quickly than whole oats. While whole oats, have a nuttier taste and a chewier texture, cooked rolled oats are very soft and mush easily.

Whole oats, because they are chewier than rolled oats, are ideal for adding bulk to vegetarian burgers. You can also add a spoon or two to your fruit smoothie before blending to thicken and boost fiber.

Water

We humans, like Mother Earth, are made of 70% water. The amount of water you need to drink depends on how much raw food you eat which contains natural waters and how active you are. The rule of thumb is to take your body weight and divide it an half, this number represents the number of ounces of water you need to drink to hydrate your bodily tissues.

Another indicator to know if you are drinking enough water is by your urine color and odor. When you are properly hydrated your urine is light yellow and odorless. The more dehydrated you are the darker your urine is and the stronger the odor gets.

When you are detoxing you need additional water, beyond the maintenance amount, to push through the extra fiber and flush out the toxins you are stirring up. Do not skimp on water and liquids when detoxing or you will be ill.

Infrared Sauna

Unlike traditional saunas that use air and steam, infrared saunas emit a radiant heat that is absorbed directly into the body. This makes it much more efficient in removing toxins with an estimated 80% water and 20% waste and toxin removal, as opposed to 97% water and 3% waste and toxins in a traditional steam sauna.

Infrared saunas are non-invasive and can penetrate as much as 3 inches into the body, which heats muscle tissue and internal organs. This will help eliminate all kinds of toxins including medications, alcohol, nicotine, and other carcinogens in the bloodstream.

Not only that, but eliminating these toxins through the skin generally creates way less symptoms that it might if it had to go through all the different detoxification pathways internally.

If you feel like you are on the verge of getting sick, popping into an infrared sauna for 15-20 minutes each day can help you knock it down before it decides to take over. The radiant heat will stimulate circulation, increase the production of white blood cells, and stimulate your immune system to mount a vigorous attack against unwanted invaders. All of this action will create a less than hospitable environment for germs to grow, and encourage them to die off.

After all, the body's natural mechanism to fight off invasive microbes is to "heat up" by creating what we call a fever. This is simply a way to help facilitate the same type of reaction, without all the unpleasant symptoms that often come with a fever.

Rebounding

Get on a trampoline or rebounder for 5-10 minutes each day. The bouncing helps pump and decongest the lymphatic fluid in the entire body. It's a simple but profound way to support the lymphatic system. The lymphatic system, a system of lymph fluid and lymph nodes, is vital for detoxification. The lymphatic system can be aptly described as the garbage disposal of the body and is responsible for filtering and eliminating toxins. The lymph nodes house a high concentration of white blood cells that increase when the body is fighting off illness or infection.

The most important thing to remember about the lymphatic system is that it relies on our body's movement. Unlike the cardiovascular system with the heart automatically pumping fluid, the lymph system relies on our body movements as a pump. Inactivity is the worst thing for lymphatic flow.

Dry Skin Brushing

The lymphatic system is pretty close to the surface of the skin. It doesn't take deep pressure to help release lymphatic congestion, which is why dry brushing your skin is so helpful. This process requires just a few minutes before your shower and stimulates lymphatic flow. You simply brush your body with a stiff, natural bristle dry brush and this activates the lymphatic system.

The mechanical action of dry brushing is wonderful for exfoliating dry winter skin. It also helps detoxify by increasing blood circulation and promoting lymph flow/drainage. Dry brushing unclogs pores in the exfoliation process. It also stimulates your nervous system, which can make you feel invigorated afterward.

Dry brushing is exactly what it sounds like, brushing your dry, not wet, skin with a dry brush. The technique is incredibly simple: Using a natural bristled dry brush, brush your whole body gently in large strokes towards the heart. Yes, that's it!

Dry skin brushing is essentially a dry massage to help prevent as well as help heal illnesses of all kinds. It is traditional to the Ayurvedic practice of medicine with historical roots in India from more than 5,000 years ago. The technique that has also been used for centuries by Scandinavians, Turks, and Russians to eliminate impurities and toxins and maintain healthy skin.

Detox Baths

The beauty of a detox bath is that you can take it whenever you want and whenever you feel like you need one.

- A hot bath can help to open your pores and get you to sweat, which may help the detoxifying process slightly.
- Hot water also helps dissolve the oils, salts and clays you may be adding in the water.
- Hot water can also be very relaxing, so that's why it's recommended for detox baths.

Pain and Stress Detox Bath

Add the following to hot bath water:

- 2 cups Epsom salt; magnesium has over 400 functions in the body
- ½ cup baking soda; detox's, changes pH, reduces swelling
- 10 drops essential oil of your liking

Soak and repeat throughout your detox as necessary.

Release Trapped Emotions

The Detoxification process occurs on a physical, spiritual and emotional level and can help uncover and express feelings, especially hidden frustrations, anger, resentments, or fear. Often, the more toxins a person releases, the more stored emotion that is also released. Dr. Dietrich Klinghardt noticed this pattern in his work with thousands of chronically ill patients and noted that "for each unresolved psycho-emotional conflict or trauma there is an equivalent of stored toxins and an equivalent of pathogenic microorganisms. To successfully detoxify the body the three issues have to be addressed simultaneously." It is important that these emotions are allowed to be processed and released to avoid causing additional stress that would undermine the detoxification process. The liver holds onto traumatic experiences and negative emotions, like anger, impatience, resentment and frustration creating emotional blocks which cause the liver to become sluggish. Processing and releasing these negative emotions are an important step in opening the drainage pathways.

Detoxification Pathways

Your ability to detoxify heavy metals, environmental toxins, bacteria, viruses and fungi is critical to your health. Any build-up of these pathogens in the body keeps your immune system on high alert and triggers chronic inflammation, both of which interfere with your ability to heal.

In order to leave your body, toxins or pathogens flow from the cell to the lymphatic fluid where they are carried into the blood, processed through the liver, then eliminated via the gall bladder carrying them to the intestines in the bile where they are eliminated with your bowel movements.

Any congestion or stagnation in these detoxification pathways can compromise your ability to detoxify.

Lymphatic System

The lymphatic system is critical for moving metabolic waste, toxins and infections out of the cells via the lymphatic fluid. It serves a dual role as a detoxification pathway and an important part of the immune system through the lining in the gut, which is 80% of our immune system. Interstitial lymph fluid permeates every part of the body and flows through the lymph nodes where toxins are filtered out, acting as a pre-filter for the liver to prevent clogging and liver overload. The lymphatic system also helps carry nutrients, oxygen, hormones and other healing substances into every cell. Unfortunately, the lymphatic system doesn't have a pump and lymphatic fluid can accumulate and stagnate. This stagnation can be due to an overload of acidity, animal protein, gluten, infection, toxins or adhesions of the connective tissue, such as scars.

The more you can help the lymph fluid flow, the more quickly you can move toxins out of the body. This is why saunas, dry brushing and jumping on a trampoline are recommended.

Intestines

Our intestines are critical for both physically breaking down our food, so we can digest, absorb and assimilate the nutrients and also eliminating the waste. Regular and healthy bowel movements are a critical pathway for the toxins to leave the body. Poor waste elimination is often correlated with toxins being reabsorbed into the body, often known as re-toxification.

The intestines also play an important role in our detoxification and immune health, providing a physical barrier to stop viruses, bacteria, fungus, yeast, parasites and other pathogens or toxins from entering the body and maintaining a balance of "good" bacteria that assist in the detoxification of toxins and the maintenance of a balanced gut environment. Normal detoxification during digestion depends on the integrity of the GI membrane and the maintenance of the precise bacterial and chemical environment. An imbalance in the intestinal flora and injury to intestinal walls, can allow undigested food and other contaminants to leak into the bloodstream.

Skin

The skin is our largest organ and a major elimination pathway. Our sweat glands act as a key channel helping to support any toxic overflow from the liver or kidneys. For example, skin reactions like acne, rosacea, psoriasis or rashes are often an indication that the liver and kidneys are processing more toxins than the body can handle, so your pores will start to pitch in to sweat things out.

Sweat therapy can trace its roots to Native American sweat lodges, Roman baths, Scandinavian saunas, and Turkish baths and recent research corroborates the benefits, finding toxins like heavy metals in sweat post exercise. Fat soluble toxins, such as endocrine disruptors like BPA, can also escape via in the sweat as well. Supporting the detoxification pathway via the skin can lessen the burden on other detox organs like the liver and the kidneys (which is especially helpful for the kidneys as they are delicate organs and can be easily damaged by overuse).

Kidneys

The kidneys are two bean-shaped organs that filter blood and remove water-soluble waste products. The kidneys also regulate the balance of fluids in the body, blood pressure (by maintaining the salt and water balance) and the body's acid-alkaline balance (pH) by selectively filtering out or retaining various minerals and electrolytes.

The kidneys are small organs but they process about 20% of the entire amount of blood pumped out by the heart. As a result, they process about 200 quarts of blood every day in an effort to filter out waste products and extra water. This processed blood is returned to the body and the eliminated waste stays in the urine and is stored in the bladder until it is excreted from the body through the urethra. Due to the heavy amount of work this tiny organ does, we need to keep it working effectively and efficiently. They control the volume, composition and pressure of fluids in all the cells. Blood flows through the kidneys at its highest pressure, filtering out toxins and directing nourishing materials to where they are needed. It is important to support the detoxification pathway of the kidneys because when the kidneys are overburdened, it will impair other detoxification channels.

The kidneys can also hold onto feelings of fear, insecurity, aloof, isolated and paranoia which can impair function. In Chinese medicine, the kidneys are considered the seat of courage and willpower. Water is symbolic of the unconscious, our emotion and of that which we do not understand and that which we fear.

Lungs

The lungs are sponge-like organs located near the backbone on either side of the heart. They serve as a fundamental source of life energy transporting oxygen from the atmosphere into the capillaries so they can oxygenate blood as well as an important channel of elimination releasing carbon dioxide from the bloodstream into the atmosphere.

Our lungs inhale and exhale an average of 16,000 times a day. Optimal lung function, and effectiveness as a detoxification pathway can be challenged by outdoor and indoor air pollution and poor lifestyle habits (smoking, lack of exercise, shallow breathing).

Similarly, emotions like feelings of grief, bereavement, regret, loss, remorse can obstruct ability of the lungs to accept and relinquish, impeding their function of "taking in" and "letting go". Grief that remains unresolved can become chronic and create disharmony in the lungs, weakening the lung's function of circulating oxygen around the body.

When lung function is impaired, it leads to shortness of breath, fatigue and feelings of melancholy.

Liver

Our liver is the largest solid organ in our bodies. It is the size of a football and weighs around 3 pounds. It takes the brunt of our poor diet and lifestyle choices including chemically treated, processed and GMO foods, toxic personal care products, prescription drugs, heavy metal poisoning, treated water, over consumption of sugar, and much more.

The liver is responsible for filtering the blood from toxins and helps eliminate any toxins that do get into the blood stream. Without it, we would become a toxic cesspool and would succumb to the toxic overload quite quickly. So it makes sense that we keep this humble working organ as healthy as possible so it can remain our best detoxification pathway.

Liver stress symptoms include sensitivity to smells (smoke, perfume, etc.) and or chemicals or those who are easily intoxicated or hung over.

Emotions held in the liver; anger, resentment, frustration, irritability, bitterness, and "flying off the handle".

Spleen

The spleen, located in the left upper quadrant of the abdomen, assists with the distribution of healthy blood cells, filtering and storing our blood in much the same way as the lymph nodes filter lymph fluid. Our blood is very sensitive to, and easily effect by, toxins. Once infiltrated with toxins, the blood can become a shuttle and depository for the toxins. This is why the spleen, while technically part of the lymphatic system, serves as an important detoxification pathway, that must be supported in any detoxification effort.

Just like the liver, the spleen recognizes and removes old, malformed, or damaged cells from the blood and helps fight off infection. For example, the lymphocytes in the spleen help destroy any toxins or pathogens in the blood. Macrophages in the spleen then help clean up any remaining debris.

The spleen is a highly vascular organ, containing many vessels that carry and circulate fluids in your body and is highly susceptible to stagnation. According to Chinese medicine, the spleen houses the body's thoughts and intentions and is responsible for analytical thinking, memory, cognition, intelligence, and ideas. These emotions in their extreme states, over-thinking, worry, excessive mental and intellectual stimulation or any activity that involves a lot of mental effort can contribute to disharmony and stagnation in the spleen. If you "ruminate" and obsess constantly about life experiences, you literally are not "transforming" them into positive fuel to motivate taking action and moving forward in life.

CHAPTER 16

Protect Yourself From Chemicals and Heavy Metals

"Water and air, the two essential fluids on which all life depends, have become global garbage cans." Jacques-Yves Cousteau

According to the United States Dept. of Labor, "Toxic metals, including "heavy metals," are individual metals and metal compounds that negatively affect people's health." Even still, heavy metals are present in nearly all aspects of modern life.

- Iron may be the most common as it accounts for 90% of all refined metals.
- Platinum may be the most universal given it is said to be found in, or used to produce, 20% of all consumer goods.
- Chromium, arsenic, cadmium, mercury, and lead have the greatest potential to cause harm on account of their extensive use.
- Mercury may be considered the worst due to its ever-present potency in fish, water and even vaccines.

Man-made chemicals are not natural to the earth, they were never meant to be in our bodies. Humans, animals and Mother Earth are being stressed, diseased and killed because of them.

Environmental chemicals are neurotoxins and hormone disrupters causing lower testosterone, infertility, miscarriages, lower IQs, autism, behavior disorders, parkinsons, breast cancer, early puberty, and more.

Chemical companies lobby government officials to the point regulatory agencies dismiss the science that proves we are being involuntarily poisoned. Chemicals have more legal rights than humans.

The Invasive Approach to Beauty

Women have such pressure to always look pretty. Outer beauty is highly sought after but the truth is beauty has a short shelf life and if you aren't cultivating your true feminine radiance your beauty will fade. But your true divine feminine radiance can and will continue to shine no matter what age you are. Yes, there's botox and other anti-aging procedures, but you can only hold back the process of aging for so long. It's ultimately all from within.

Conventional Anti-aging treatments include a long list of tedious and elaborate processes. The most common ones include Botox, Facelift, Necklift, Eye Bag removal, fat injections, and anti-aging creams. Most of the inexpensive creams contain toxic ingredients like:

- Sodium Lauryl Sulfate (SLS)
- Acrylamide
- Propylene glycol (PEG)
- Phenol carbolic acid
- Toluene
- Alcohols

- DEA (diethanolamine)
- MEA (monoethanolamine)
- TEA (triethanolamine)
- Nitrosamines
- Padimate-O
- Triclosan

Sodium Lauryl Sulfate (SLS) is one of the most common ingredients found in over 90% of anti-aging wrinkle creams. SLS can reduce the level of moisture in your skin and lead to skin dryness with early signs of aging. SLS has an ability to combine with other chemicals to form "nitrosamine", which is a potent carcinogen.

Phenol carbolic acid may lead to convulsions, coma, circulatory collapse, paralysis and even death from respiratory failure. Usage of toluene by pregnant women may affect a developing fetus. Toluene is found in most synthetic fragrances and is obtained from coal tar or petroleum. One must remember that every toxic substance applied on the surface of the skin gets absorbed by your body and may lead to grave consequences including skin cancer, skin irritation and other associated risks.

26 seconds is all it takes for chemicals from your personal care products to enter your blood stream.

What You Can Do: As horrifying as all this is we still want to look beautiful and as young as possible for as long as possible. Experiment with the many natural ingredient products until you find what you like and what works for you. There are more coming on the market as demand rises and there are also many DIY lotions, creams, oils, soaps, deodorants, perfumes and shampoos available in books and online.

The Natural Approach to Beauty

A holistic approach aimed at the physical and energetic root causes of aging, is necessary to age gracefully.

What You Can Do:

- Supply your body with essential vitamins, minerals and nutrients which are depleted due to aging.
- Restore impaired metabolism.
- Correct the digestive and assimilative processes that deteriorate due to aging.
- Use ingredients with natural anti-oxidant properties to help combat free-radicals in your body.
- Improve energy levels, so that you may stay active and fit.
- Drink more water to hydrate your skin from the inside out.

Cosmetic and Beauty Products

Parabens, sodium laurel sulfates, diethanolamine are a few of the harmful chemicals used in our personal care products. From conditioners and shampoos to makeup and perfumes, facial moisturizers and body lotions, toothpaste and mouthwash, bath soap and hand sanitizers, nail polish and polish remover, gel and acrylic nails, hairspray and hair dye, antiperspirants and deodorants. These chemicals introduce harmful toxins into your bloodstream through the skin.

What You Can Do: We might be absorbing several pounds of chemicals through the makeup, lotions and other items we use on a daily basis. We must always check to see the ingredients used. Avoid those with things like talc, lanolin and phthalates. Also, avoid the use of body care products that have synthetic colors and limit your use of non-natural perfumes. Brush with a fluoride-free toothpaste or powder.

Cleaning and Home Products

There are hundreds of chemicals in laundry soap and fabric softeners, dish soaps and scrubbers, toilet and shower scrubs, carpet cleaners, bleaches and antiseptic soaps and wipes, window and car wash cleaners, spray air fresheners, plug in and hanging air fresheners, candles, fabric and carpet sprays, paint and varnishes.

These products can cause rashes, allergies, respiratory problems and cancer. Bleach based, Ammonia based products that are found in our homes for cleaning purposes and killing germs are a serious danger to our health.

What You Can Do: Try Eliminating all Toxic cleaning products from you home. The best product to use for cleaning your home is soap and water. Baking soda work very well at disinfecting and scrubbing without the dangerous side effects.

Use organic, natural, biodegradable products such as white vinegar and essential oils. Choose carefully and read labels when purchasing products and make your own when possible. You will not only be healthier but save money.

Pots and Pans

Nonstick cookware has been a real time saver in our kitchens. Unfortunately there's some serious health concerns associated with Teflon and in particular a chemical that it releases in certain conditions called PFOA. PFOA and other chemicals in Teflon coatings have been labeled as 'likely to be carcinogenic to humans' by a panel reporting to the Environmental Protection Agency.

2010 research found higher blood levels of PFOA to be associated with a greater risk of thyroid disease, a serious health issue that has skyrocketed in recent years. Studies have also linked exposure to the chemical to a higher risk of heart disease and stroke, even at relatively low levels.

High-temperature cooking with these type of pans can lead to a condition known as 'Teflon flu' from inhaling the gases released over your hot plate.

Symptoms of Teflon flu are actually said to be quite similar to suddenly developing influenza, with headaches, chills and fever, along with coughing and chest tightness most commonly reported.

Because Teflon flu usually develop several hours after exposure to off-gassing nonstick pans, very few people would make the association. The temperatures involved are relatively high at above 500 degrees Fahrenheit (260 Celsius), but not that difficult to reach if heating a pan up to sear a steak in for instance.

These kind of temperatures aren't that hard to reach if you leave a pan on the hot plate for a while or heat it up on a high setting. Contrary to popular belief, you don't actually have to use metal utensils on your nonstick cookware for it to be dangerous regardless of whether your frying pan or saucepan is chipped or scratched.

While you may not have experienced such extreme symptoms, PFOA is a very persistent chemical and once in your body it is difficult to get rid of and builds up over time. Estimates of 98% of the US population having detectable levels of PFOA show just how pervasive this chemical is. Given that, it's far better to start reducing your exposure from your pots and pans today.

While its use is slowly being phased out, unless you've recently purchased cookware that is specifically labeled PFOA-free, then it's likely that the nonstick pans in your kitchen are a source of this potentially dangerous chemical.

What You Can Do: Trade In Your Teflon. This is very difficult as most of the cookware is made of Teflon. Substitute this cookware with stainless steel or baked enamel or porcelain interiors, which do not stick and cook food wonderfully, or seasoned cast iron skillets.

Food

Chemicals contaminate our food supply, blocking the natural processes of the human body. These chemicals not only cause major health issues but also make it very difficult to lose weight. Many people feel that they have become too busy to cook healthy fresh meals and rely on convenient package products like canned, boxed and processed meals which are loaded with chemical additives, food coloring, preservatives, flavor enhancers and aromas.

The people, who are supposed to be looking out for our health interest, are paid to look the other way and make false or incomplete research to assure the public their food products are safe. Companies care about profit, cheaper ingredients, and a longer shelf life. There are more than 3,000 food chemicals purposely added to our food to make it look, smell, and taste better. More chemicals are invented every day and new 'good looking' names made up for old ones.

The U.S. alone goes through roughly 1 billion pounds of pesticides each year, and these are used on healthy items like apples, strawberries, broccoli and more. These pesticides have been linked to everything from emotional instability and muscle cramps to changes in heart rate and cancer.

The lining inside the canned food products are extremely dangerous for us because of the high level of Bisphenol A, this is a commonly used ingredient found in can goods, plastic goods and is very bad for the human body. You can eliminate some of this toxin from your body by not using food stored in cans or plastic containers.

Always choose stove cooked foods instead of food that has been prepared in the Microwave; it is healthier for you and tastes much better.

What You Can Do: Dump processed foods and embrace organic whole foods instead. Choose organic foods that are raised without pesticides, herbicides, antibiotics, hormones and chemical fertilizers.

Once you switch to all organic food it only takes 6 days to detox the chemicals from the toxic food you have been eating.

Pet Food

Don't feed your beloved pet cheap food, many of which get recalls for harmful ingredients that can make them ill and even kill them. Dogs and cats in the wild eat raw wild food, they aren't meant to eat dry processed food any more than you are. They also need clean drinking water.

Dogs and cats are being diagnosed with the same health issues as humans, because of their diet and the cost of their care at the vet is as expensive as humans without insurance.

What You Can Do: Buy or make their food that has healthy meats not byproducts. Feed them fruits and vegetables and include some raw food in their diet. Stay away from fillers such as wheat and rice. Don't spray your lawn with toxic chemicals, it causes cancer in your precious pets who play on it.

Water

Six to ten glasses of pure water each day are necessary to enhance your body's functioning. Over half of your body is made up of water. It's in every cell and every tissue. Biological processes like circulation, digestion, absorption and excretion depend on water. It forms the foundation of blood and lymph, maintains hearty muscles and young-looking skin, lubricates joints and organs and regulates body temperature. You can't function without it.

Research shows the average tap water contains more than 140 contaminants. Even worse, pharmaceuticals like tranquilizers, painkillers and birth control pills are also found in tap water.

Unfortunately bottled water is no better thanks to their chemical-leaching plastic containers. Look for glass or stainless steel water bottles. Glass bottles often come with silicone sleeves to prevent shattering.

Get a whole home water filter if you can or at the very least a tabletop filter. If you live on a well, get a kit for testing your water or check with your local government to see if they offer well-testing programs.

It's very important to have a filter on your shower, since the tap water in many areas may contain substances you don't want in your body such as chlorine and fluoride and heavy metals such as lead, mercury and arsenic.

These and other substances can directly move into your body through the skin and lungs into your internal environment. When you take a steaming hot shower, you breathe in the steam and your skin absorbs the equivalent of six to eight glasses of chlorinated water. A shower filter will protect your body from absorbing the chlorine.

What You Can Do: Buy the best water filters you can. The number one priority for yourself, your family and pets is filtered drinking water. There are many choices from expensive elaborate filters to simple inexpensive models.

The same is true with bath and shower filters. We have the luxury of daily hot showers that in the past were only available to royalty and the rich. But because of the poor quality of tap water in most urban communities we must filter the water in our baths and showers.

Yard and Garden

Residue can be found on the outside of your herbs and vegetables which can be washed off, but worse is that pesticides get in & stay in plant cells when absorbed through leaves and when eaten they get right to work destroying DNA/disrupting hormones. Roots bring pesticides into plants through contaminated soil and water. Canadian Study, University of Sherbrooke, 2011 results showed 96% of unborn babies to have Bt Toxins in their blood. Pesticides are the number 1 reason for birth defects/lower IQ.

What You Can Do: Purchase or make your own organic fertilizers, herbicides and pesticides for your lawn and home gardens. There are many recipes and formulas online that are very easy to make.

Lawns

Schools, homes and parks are routinely sprayed with herbicides and pesticides causing allergies and cancer in kids, dogs and lawn care workers. There are currently law suites against Round Up, the most used brand around the world and it is slowly being banned.

What You Can Do: Do not use these poisons in and around your home and protest the use of them in our schools and parks. There are many natural options that an be used to control weeds and insects such as white vinegar, dish soap, borax, table salt, boiling water, neem oil, diatomaceous earth, garlic and pepper spray.

Plastics

Plastic affects human health. Plastic water bottles and food storage containers, plastic wraps, plastic microwave containers, etc. have a negative affect on the human body. Toxic chemicals leach out of plastic and are found in the blood and tissue of nearly all of us. Exposure to them is linked to cancers, birth defects, impaired immunity, endocrine disruption and other ailments.

What You Can Do: Throw out all plastics which contain bisphenol-A (BPA), PVC or Phthalates. Replace those plastic items with alternatives like items made from safe plastics, glass, steel, ceramics, wood or cloth.

How To Makes Changes In Your Life As You've Always Known It

All of the above information is a lot to take in and requires many changes and a different mindset. There are a few who are "all or nothing" and can instantly make changes in their life but for most of us it is a little more challenging.

I suggest you make a list of all the changes you want to make, then put them in order from the easiest to the hardest.

Begin with the item which is the easiest to change, conquer it and mark it off your list then go on the next easiest, working your way down the list to the hardest. By then your changes will be easier to make as your resolve is stronger.

When you begin with the easiest change you are much more likely to continue your desired lifestyle changes than those who begin with the item they feel is the most important but may also be the most difficult change and they eventually give up on the whole idea.

By making these mindful changes you will significantly decrease the chances of you, your family and pets developing any life threatening disease.

CHAPTER 17

Sacred Pregnancy

The Female Being has been chosen by the Creator to be the portal between the spiritual realm and this physical realm. She is the only force on earth powerful enough to navigate unborn spirits onto this planet.

The Divine Feminine is an extremely powerful force within us. It has characteristics that we associate with mothering: it helps you grow, it helps you create, it cultivates who you are. One of the reasons we give the Earth the title of "Mother Earth" is because of the Divine Feminine.

Everything grows on Earth. She feeds you, holds you, cares for you and supports you. The caretakers among us know it requires a lot of strength and energy to do that. The Divine Feminine is all about the associations we have with a nurturing mother.

All over the world, for the hundreds of thousands of years we have been the divine feminine giving birth, which has been a very risky business. Until 100 years ago, 1 in 10 women died in childbirth. Of all the ways women met their death, giving birth was one of the most common. If they survived a difficult birth, they were often left weakened and anemic with trauma to their pelvic tissues. If their babies survived, they needed to successfully breast-feed, as there was no formula for babies. Mothers who found themselves barely alive had to also provide the milk for their babies to survive.

In indigenous and ancient times babies were delivered and moms were tended to by a midwife and female family members. The birthing of babies was a divine feminine undertaking. A shaman, medicine man or doctor was only called to assist in emergencies.

For much of human history, pregnancy and childbirth was an extremely dangerous period in a woman's life. It was often believed that the expectant mother and her baby were vulnerable to malevolent supernatural forces. Therefore, many ancient civilizations developed childbirth rituals which were believed to protect both the mother and her baby from harm. As it was believed that evil spirits would attack a woman while she was giving birth, many ancient societies had a deity or several deities who would be given the task of protecting women in labor.

Having had three child births myself, I can tell you when you are in hard labor the things you do and say could easily look to others like you are possessed and it feels more like you are being attacked by evil spirits than it does a spiritual experience!

It isn't until it is all over you can appreciate the miracle and honor it is to bring a new little human into the world and to acknowledge your power as a co-creator in the spiritual realm.

Prepare Your Body Before Pregnancy

Good nutrition is most important immediately prior to conception and during the first 12 weeks of pregnancy (including the very early stages, when the woman is unaware she is pregnant). It is therefore important for women to maintain a healthy diet throughout their childbearing years, and particularly if they are planning to become pregnant.

A woman's nutritional status during pregnancy depends on the availability of her nutritional reserves of particular micro-nutrients such as calcium and iron, which have been built up in her body from prior consumption of foods containing those micro-nutrients. As these reserves build up before a woman becomes pregnant, maintaining good nutrition prior to conception is vital for ensuring adequate nutritional status during pregnancy. Women who are underweight or overweight, or who have deficiencies in particular micro-nutrients rarely "catch-up" by improving their diet once they are pregnant, as at this stage their body already faces additional nutritional demands because of the growing baby.

Obviously quit alcohol, smoking and drugs. Alcohol, smoke and drug abuse may turn your pregnancy disastrous. It is recommended to quit these habits much before conception as they apparently cause birth defects in the child and often cause intra uterine deaths as well. Seek assistance to quit these habits to have a healthy baby.

Your oral health condition speaks volumes about your overall health and the inconsistency in your hormones in pregnancy may cause bleeding and swelling gums. It is important to keep monitoring your oral health before and during pregnancy.

Studies revealed that women need to take B vitamin throughout the pregnancy and at least once a month before pregnancy as this vitamin helps preventing massive birth defects related to the spine and brain of the babies. Dark green leafy veggies are natural sources of folic acid. Fortified whole grains and cereals and citrus fruits are also good sources to this prenatal vitamin.

Adolescents and teenagers tend to be fussy eaters unless they make the meal themselves. They should be taught healthy eating habits and how to prepare meals at a young age to help them care for themselves. Young girls should be taught the importance of keeping their bodies healthy and strong, not just for themselves but also for future pregnancies, long before they plan for or accidently become pregnant.

After Delivery

We certainly should celebrate the birth of a new citizen of the planet, and the woman who put her body and her life at risk to accomplish this miracle.

Long ago the resting period after delivery in the US was anywhere from two weeks to two months, even for healthy woman, it was their confinement and recuperation time. Of course, this was the luxury for woman of some financial means. Many women in the 1800s had no choice but to get up shortly after birth, and take care of the baby, all the other children, and help out on the farm. Although, most women were attended by other women in their family, or church community, and hopefully, a skilled birth attendant, they didn't have two weeks or two months to stay in bed.

Until World War I and World War II, women who gave birth in a hospital stayed in bed at the hospital for a week or two, recovering from the delivery. When hospital beds were needed for wounded soldiers, the time in the hospital was decreased from two weeks to one week, to four days, to our present 48 hours.

Women are often exhausted and beat up after the birth of a child, especially the first one, they're often bruised, and battered down there. Their bladders don't work and their hemorrhoids hurt. Breast-feeding every two hours doesn't help with the sleep problems. About 70 percent of women have the baby blues in the first couple weeks postpartum, and about five percent of women will develop postpartum depression.

The first two weeks are rocky. That's the time that moms are establishing their milk production and their feeding schedule.

They need to drink a lot of fluids, and eat a balanced diet of whole grains, lots of fiber for that beat up bum, fruits, vegetables, and protein. They may continue taking their prenatal vitamins several weeks for nutritional replacement and if they had significant blood loss, iron rich foods or iron replacement may be recommended.

New mothers need a lot of rest. But as soon as they're comfortable they need to get up and walk around. This is important for decreasing the risk of blood clots. Family can help by taking on the cooking and cleaning responsibilities in the home for the first two weeks or maybe the first two months. It is beneficial for the mother and newborn avoiding strenuous physical activity and restricting visitors to allow recuperation and reduce risk for infections.

Too many new mothers rush back to their daily routines after birth. They expect that their weight, energy levels, mood and libido will miraculously bounce back without any assistance; they also believe it is normal for their bodies to feel wrecked from childbearing. Some modern mothers never fully recover from having children. Instead, they suffer from depression, lack of libido, weight gain, hormonal imbalances, inability to conceive more children, urinary incontinence and other complications.

Belly Binding

Abdominal binders have been used for centuries after the birth of a baby. The goal for this postpartum tool is to help a new mother feel more stable, be able to get around more easily and to improve her posture.

Binding is a roll of stretchy cloth for a new mother to wrap around her abdomen, minimize organ prolapse, improve the waistline and return internal organs to the correct position.

For centuries, women around the world have practiced the unique post-pregnancy binding in an effort to prevent hip widening. It is believed that snugly binding the hips right after pregnancy help the loosened pelvic joints stabilize and returns the hips to their pre-pregnancy width. Tightly binding the hips effectively reduces the circumference of the pelvic bones.

The binding method must be done within 8 weeks after giving birth when the hormone Relaxin is still circulating in high levels in the mother's system. The hormone helps the joints and ligaments remain loose so that the binding the joints returns them to their pre-pregnancy size.

For best effects, the hips need to be bound the first week postpartum after a vaginal delivery and within 4 to 6 weeks postpartum after a cesarean section. The binding will continue for ten hours per day for at least 40 days. Don't wear them too tight or too long.

Spacing Babies

Children born at least three but less than five years apart are the healthiest children with fewer complications, defects and deaths. Women should wait at least 24 months before conceiving their next child for their own health and well-being. This is especially important for women who have had multiple deliveries, twins and triplets, which placed a greater demand on her body.

Too many women have already had intercourse before their 6 week checkup following delivery and many don't wait the minimum time of 18 months before getting pregnant again, which puts a great burden on her body. This is not enough time for her to recover and build up her reserves of nutrients for the next child. This is a very bad practice given we live in a society with increasing autism, adhd, mental illness, birth defects and postpartum depression.

Benefits of Healthy Birth Spacing:

- Baby can develop well because Mom can give lots of attention to the baby.
- Mom will have more energy and be less "stressed out".
- Mom will have more time to bond with the baby.
- Future babies will be healthier because Mom's body had enough time to replace nutrient stores before getting pregnant again.
- Children who are adequately spaced are better prepared to begin kindergarten, and perform better in school.
- Mom has more time to spend with the child and the child receives more attention and assistance with developmental tasks.
- Families have more time to bond with each child.
- Parents have more time for each other.
- Parents can have time to themselves.
- Families can have less financial stress.

Be unapologetic about the Divine Feminine you are and the value you add to the world. Make extreme self-care a high priority so you can joyfully take care of the new beings you bring into the world.

CHAPTER 18

Extreme Self-Care is the Pathway to Divine Feminine Wellness

You can't transform your health and be radiant on top of a belief that other people's needs have a higher priority than your own.

Extreme self-care is taking care of your body, mind, heart and spirit. It is about loving yourself and others. It is about doing things that you enjoy and standing up for things you think are right and serving others. Extreme self-care is living a purposeful life and standing in your Divine Femininity.

Tuning into the Divine Feminine will lead you to your path of wholeness and make the connection between body, mind, heart and spirit which will help you be your best, brightest self, and live a healthier, more joyful life.

Another overarching principle of wholeness is that we are the ultimate healers of ourselves. We need to be at the forefront of supporting ourselves because all external help is just secondary.

We have become too sophisticated as a people and that is one of our down falls. We need to get back to primitive godliness and simplicity if we wish to regain our peace and happiness.

We need to relearn what our ancient ancestors knew about spending time in nature, living in community, using plants for food and medicine and recognize energy and spiritual healing as bonafide therapy. Our DNA recognizes the ancient remedies and responds with health and happiness.

Healing Your Whole Being

Our bodies are made of and supported by nature and therefore can only be healed by nature in the long term. Chemicals are often necessary for immediate change in an acute situation but tend to do the body more harm than good in the long run. One would use wood to fix a desk made of wood or metal to fix a car made of metal, so why use chemicals to fix a body made of nature?

Each human is a child of immortality pre-programmed to perform a billion functions with a mind boggling precision that most science cannot comprehend. Life cannot be recreated with chemical interactions and there is much more to life than molecular interactions. Our bodies are the most advanced pharmacies on the planet and millions of functions happen each minute with astounding precision.

Nature has blessed the Earth with natural medicines and healing mechanisms. It would be wise not to ignore them. The intelligence of nature is much greater than that of man. Unfortunately, man still focuses on chemical medicines, as they can be patented and sold for huge profits.

Homeopathic and Naturopathic methods are never studied and verified by governing bodies, as there is no one who will spend millions obtaining an approval on herbs, knowing that they cannot be patented and sold exclusively by them. Modern man who wants scientific proof of everything ignorantly discards these methods of healing as quackery.

True healing addresses the physical, energetic, mental and emotional layers of your being. Every thought, emotion, vibration or action leads to a series of chemical changes in the body. All ailments are a result of disharmony in the life force. Holistic healing is necessary for lasting relief.

Treating an ailment on the molecular level alone, seldom has a lasting effect as the untreated social, emotional, mental, spiritual and energetic patterns will cause the ailment to manifest once again on a physical plane.

Good health involves every aspect of our being including diet, lifestyle, exercise, emotional states, thoughts and energetic patterns. Emotions and physical health are intimately connected. Emotional imbalances can act as both symptoms and causes for physical issues. Additionally, mental health conditions are linked to specific ailments of key organs.

Mental Healing

Mental healing is focused on eliminating all deep-seated thoughts that make us ill. When we are psychologically distressed, our bodies will surely manifest through restlessness, fatigue and even serious diseases. This is why we must put emphasis on the importance of mind healing.

Healing your mind does not simply mean thinking positively. It goes beyond just shifting your thoughts. Mental healing is all about creating healthy thinking patterns that you will follow every single day. It's claiming back the power over your mind and controlling it to your advantage. One of the challenges of having a physical body is leaning to control the mind.

One simple way of programming your mind is through self-talk. Incorporating the habit of affirming yourself to your everyday routine works wonders for your overall mental healing. Know that the way you talk to yourself shapes the way you perceive yourself. It's bridging the gap between your external sense of self and your core, your soul. So make sure to train yourself to speak to your mind in a kind, nurturing language.

Mental healing includes making time for yourself. Your alone time when you can think, plan, journal, nap, meditate and pray without interruptions. Everyone needs and deserves time alone for their peace of mind and sanity.

Spiritual Healing

Soul healing focuses on nurturing your spiritual health by "feeding" it. This could mean by engaging in spiritual activities, praying, or consuming materials like spiritual books or podcasts. Your soul is your core. This is one of the reasons why you may feel that sometimes, it can be out of reach. It takes a special, guided approach to be able to speak to your soul, as it houses your deepest feelings.

This is where meditation healing comes into the picture. Meditation, when done properly, creates a gateway between our external selves and our soul. When we meditate, the direct spiritual connection that we create allows us to get a hold of our soul and heal it faster.

We are all guilty of disregarding our spiritual health. We think that only the body can get wounded, as the soul is intangible to us. Spiritual healing pulls us back from this belief. When we embark on a journey of spiritual cleansing, we realize that the reason why we cannot attain the highest form of well-being is because we are disconnected from the Divine.

The worst thing we ever did was put God up in the sky, beyond our reach and understanding, separating us from our source. Spiritual healing is all about reconnecting with the Divine. This also means reconnecting with nature, with people, and with our own selves. This is a holistic approach where we treat the body and soul as one and complementary, remembering we are not a body, we are a soul with a body.

"The distance between our surface world and the world of spirits is exactly as wide as the edge of a maple leaf". Handsome Lake, Seneca prophet of the Iroquois

Physical Healing

Use food as your medicine. Use herbs and plants as your medicine. Homeopathy harmonizes the entire being; flower essences attunes the mind; herbs balance the terrain of the body; vibrational and energetic therapies potentially help bring balance to the whole being. Healing the physical body is the beginning of getting to the root of healing the whole being.

Holistic Healing

The main concept behind Mind, Body, Spirit is that we are more than just our thoughts. We are also our bodies, our emotions, and our spirituality, all these things combine to give us identity, determine our health, and make us who we are.

Holistic healing is the amalgamation of all types of healing. Founded in the philosophy of a unified being, holistic considers the body, the mind, the heart and the soul. This means that we cannot achieve the highest form of healing if we just focus on treating only one part of our being. Notice that all of the approaches in this book target not just a certain area of the body but the entire psyche. Holistic healing aims to restore the balance of the overall health of the whole divine being.

Another overarching principle of holistic healing is that we are the ultimate healers of ourselves. We need to be at the forefront of supporting ourselves because all external help is just secondary.

Our body, mind, heart and spirit are our own responsibility and no one else's.

Holistic Health is your overall state of wellness on all levels of your being. It encompasses the health of your entire being and extends to everyone and everything that affects you in any way. That includes your resources, your environment and your relationships.

Ancient women put a special sacred meaning in everything they were doing. Cooking, embroidery towels, brushing their hair, etc. was a magical ritual. Everything that women did, they charged with their energy through their prayers and manifestations. Maybe that's why families were more harmonious and stronger, and people were healthier and happier. It's time for us to put that knowledge back into our lives, and also begin to treat our daily chores, responsibilities, and beauty care as sacred rituals.

Make Your Health a Top Priority

Your first step is to give yourself permission to take time for your own well-being. Ask yourself: Who will take care of me if I run myself into the ground? What will happen to the people I care about? It may sound counter-intuitive, but self-care is critical to taking care of others.

You can't transform your health and be radiant on top of a belief that other people's needs have a higher priority than your own.

Out of our love, concern and sense of responsibility to our loved ones and families we too often put their needs and wants before our own. You may think they will recognize your sacrifices, appreciate you and love you all the more for it, but you would be wrong. They come to expect this is how it should be, and take you for granted. You will raise entitled children and a husband who thinks he is superior to you and come to expect his needs and wants should be met before yours.

Your misguided efforts of love and sacrifice are a disservice to them. You are not teaching your daughters to honor their Divine Feminine, because you aren't being a good example of it, and for your sons and husbands you are perpetuating the old myth of male superiority and domination.

You are behaving the opposite of your true self; a sacred divine feminine, spiritual goddess, heiress to the first revered divine women on earth.

Loving yourself and self-care is not selfish, it is showing you understand who you really are. It shows respect and love to your heavenly mother and father who created you. It shows your understanding that we are all loved and important and equal in deserving our needs to be met.

Our family life is where we learn and practice on each other how we will act and relate to the outside world. As a mother and woman on a spiritual journey, the most loving thing you can do is to elevate yourself on the priority list and be an example of a divine feminine mother, wife and partner. The problem with always putting them first is you are teaching them that you come second.

If you feel you need organic food for your health, nutritional counseling, weight loss support, nutritional supplements, exercise equipment, clothes that fit you and are in current style, etc. make sure your needs are equally as important as any other family member. I am not saying you are the most important and always come first, but you are not always last either.

The next time you feel compelled to be a martyr, ask yourself "What would a Goddess do in this situation?"

Your Body Believes Everything You Tell It

If you understood the power of thoughts, belief and intention you would never have a negative thought again. Your thoughts have more power than you can imagine. There have been many books written about mind over matter, for good reason.

Jesus taught saying, "I tell you the truth, if you had faith even as small as a mustard seed, you could say to this mountain, 'Move from here to there,' and it would move. Nothing would be impossible." (Matthew 17:20)

Having power over your own body seems more manageable than moving a mountain! You are the master of your thoughts and your body. Your body is your gift, your temple, your vehicle, your responsibility. It's job is to stay alive to take you through your journey on earth. Your body loves you and wants to live for you, it knows how to heal and repair itself to stay alive as long as possible.

Your job is to love your body, take care of it and be grateful for all it has done for you and enabled you to experience as an earthly being. Have you birthed a child, climbed a mountain, snow skied or surfed ocean waves? Love your perfectly imperfect body for enabling you to experience thrilling earthly adventures. Look at your feet. Maybe they are oddly shaped but just think of the miles they have walked to carry you around this world and all of the things you have been able to do and places you have been able to go because of them.

We didn't come to earth with a handbook on how to care for our bodies because it is so simple. Modern life and western medicine has made it seem complicated and beyond our individual abilities to care for ourselves. This of course is a lie and this old belief system takes away our divine power to believe in ourselves, and the power of Mother Nature and our Creator.

Personal Power

When we feel fragile because the magnitude of life feels too heavy, sometimes the only thing we can do is focus on Extreme Feminine Self- Care. Looking after ourselves is a large aspect of building our personal power. And when we are able to access our divine internal strength, it will see us through the deeply challenging and confronting times life throws at us.

Trust your needs. Do not judge them. Allow them. Act on them. You may just find your Divine self again.

CONCLUSION

Put love and blessing in everything you do. Treat everything you do as ritual, giving it a special sacred meaning. It is in such seemingly invisible acts of a woman that her true magical power manifests itself.

Your soul lives in a physical body in order to navigate through life on earth. There is a "you" inside of you. Your body loves you, its only job is to keep you alive, at all costs. It is your willing servant. Your body has the ability to heal and repair itself to keep you alive for many years to allow you to experience your human earthly adventure.

Women are physical representatives of feminine energy on our planet. Unfortunately, most modern women have forgotten their original nature, a nature of divinity. It is time to bring ancient wisdom alive and use your Divine Feminine Energy to love, heal and nurture yourself and Mother Earth.

Extreme self-care is attending to the needs of your whole being. Modern humans have become disconnected from nature and its natural healing powers. We have lost our ancestors knowledge of plant medicine, energy medicine, the power of the mind to control the body, and the belief in divine intervention.

We live in a time with ancient wisdom at our fingertips and a multitude of ancient health and spiritual traditions from many cultures which are bursting forth in new forms for our Modern Age. We can bridge ancient wisdom and practices to match our modern sensibilities to heal ourselves once again even in our compromised world.

As our earth, water and food become more polluted we are suffering from man made diseases and succumbing to man made medicine, operations and radiation. All the medicine and all the medical doctors cannot heal a cut or regrow skin, your body does that all on its own. You can heal yourself of anything, any disease, any illness. But you have to stop doing what is making you sick in the first place, there isn't a pill for that.

We are suffering from constant noise and light pollution and unprecedented stress. Most people spend 90% of their time in buildings breathing recycled air, under artificial light, surrounded by radiation from electromagnetic frequencies from computers, cell phones, wifi, tv's, home appliances, and smart home devices. Some people can even go years without their bare feet actually touching the earth or the sun touching their skin.

Since ancient times people have respected the forces of Nature, seeing divinity in Mother Earth, the sun, the moon, in all life. I have included many of these ancient tools for you to use to protect your spiritual and mental health and the health of the temple of your Inner Goddess.

Ancient women put a special sacred meaning in everything they were doing, they charged everything with their energy through their prayers and manifestations. It's time for us to put that knowledge back into our lives, and also begin to treat our daily chores, responsibilities, and beauty care as sacred rituals.

Lasting healing comes by living a healthy lifestyle, more like our ancient ancestors lived. This is your pathway to true happiness, self-love, vibrant physical, mental, emotional and spiritual well-being.

- Self-care is recognizing you are in partnership with the physical body you exist in.
- Self-care is lovingly nurturing your body and loving it for everything it does for you.
- True self-care is free. It doesn't have to mean silk sheets, expensive retreats, products and treatments.
- Self-care could be as simple as writing down and journaling your feelings, eating fruit you love, going out to nature, getting plenty of sleep and rest, saying no to junk food, drinking clean water and taking a daily walk.
- Self-care is eating real food, drinking clean water and keeping your body moving.

Your body is designed to be self healing and self generating to keep you alive for 120 years, according to the Mayo Clinic. And it can, if you remember you are a living organic being that needs living organic whole food and clean water to do so. Science has now proven the body is more self healing than they ever thought, we don't loose all of our brain cells or stem cells as they once thought, in fact we can regenerate new neurotransmitters and stem cells in the brain under the right circumstances.

- You have the same body and DNA the prehistoric cave-woman had 200,000 years ago, evolution has not changed that.
- You have a prehistoric body living in a modern world. Your cave-woman body has survived and procreated for hundreds of thousands of years because we ate real whole food from the earth and used water and plants for medicine. Yet somehow we expect this ancient body to thrive in a world where most of what we eat and drink is not real food, but man-made, highly processed, chemical and sugar laden "food stuff" disguised as food.

- We slather hormone mimicking chemical soaps, lotions, cosmetics and perfumes all over our skin, hair and nails. Our food, water, air and soil are polluted and our homes, furniture and clothes emit poisonous chemicals. As a result we are suffering from man-made diseases, infertility, dull blemished skin, fatigue and depression.

If you are sick and tired all of the time you will not be able to fulfill your divine purpose or experience the joys and adventures you should be having on your earthly journey.

Using Extreme Feminine Self-Care, ancient wisdom, natural food and medicine will bring forth healing, repairing, and maintenance for the optimal health of your body, mind, heart and soul. And so it is.

To be continued in volume IV, Self-Reliance in a Changing World.

RESOURCES & REFERENCES

Alberto Villoldo, Grow a New Body
Andrew Kimbrell JD, Your Food and Your Planet
Bradley Nielsen, The Emotion Code
David Perlmutter MD
Dean Ornish MD
Dr. Gabriel Cousens, Conscious Eating
Dr. Gabriel Cousens, There is a Cure for Diabetes – Revised Edition
Elizabeth Lipski, Digestive Wellness
Game Changers, documentary
Jason Fong, Fasting; after Game Changers
Joel Furman MD
Joel Kahn MD
John and Ocean Robbins, Food Revolution
Michael Klapper MD
Neal Barnard MD
Peter Kelder, Ancient Secret of the Fountain of Youth
Robert O. Young, Sick and Tired?
Sally Fallon, Nourishing Traditions
Susan Bennett, The Kimchi Diet

ABOUT THE AUTHOR

Marilyn Pabon has a keen insight and understanding of the physical and spiritual aspects of being a woman. She spent over 20 years studying and practicing holistic nutrition, energy healing and all things related to natural wellness. She has always been a spiritual seeker, very intuitive, and has the gift of a very thin veil between our world and the spirit world.

While studying Shamanism and learning the first Shaman were women, led her to learning all she could about the history of women to include prehistory women. During this search she had an awakening as to the divinity of women, the divine feminine, who began the world and how their energy has returned to bring balance to the world.

With this knowledge, all of her studying and training over the years came to a full circle of understanding the big beautiful picture of the purpose and divinity of women.

Marilyn's mission is to empower women to find the path back to their souls and their divinity by guiding them toward self-love and inner transformation.

She has written a series of four books "Divine Feminine Handbook" to teach women their divine history, who they really are, their specialness, how to love themselves, have self-confidence, carry themselves like a goddess, care for their physical temples and be self sufficient.

She is a California native currently living in Utah's beautiful red rock country at the gateway to Zion National Park with her husband and daughter.

For more information about her work and books, visit: www.marilynpabon.com

SHARE THE DREAM

Divine Feminine Handbook I, II, III, and IV are more than a set of books.

It is a lifestyle and movement in which modern women can live to their greatest and truest versions of themselves. It's a dedication to empower women to break free from the shackles of outdated and limiting beliefs. It is a call to awaken the Divine Feminine Energy in us all. It is a remembrance of our divine ancient foremothers who once were revered as creators of life, healers, spiritual guides, shamans and leaders.

If you too have a dream of helping your divine sisters learn of their sacred heritage and cultivate their goddess within, so they too can live empowered fulfilling lives, please share these books.

One of the simplest ways you can do that is by leaving a review online. Write down your thoughts about the book on your favorite book selling or review sites so that other Divine Feminine women can be inspired to know more.

You can also share your ideas on your social media page. Make sure to include the official hashtag: #divinefemininehandbooks.

From my heart to yours,
Marilyn Pabon

Printed in the United States
by Baker & Taylor Publisher Services